はじめての
臨床栄養英語

清水雅子　J. パトリック バロン

English for Clinical Nutritionists

Metabolism consists of the chemical and physical processes (absorption, synthesis and decomposition of chemical substances) crucial to life of all living organisms, not just humans. After food is eaten, it is absorbed, especially in the small intestine; proteins are converted into amino acids, fats into fatty acids, and carbohydrates into simple sugars (for example glucose) by chemical digestive agents called enzymes. Blood carries these compounds with other enzymes to the cells in which two phases of metabolism, anabolism and catabolism, take place at the same time.

During anabolism, small molecules are changed into larger and more complex molecules of carbohydrate, protein and fat. Structural proteins act to repair and replace the tissue of the body. Functional proteins contain enzymes which speed up chemical reactions; antibodies which either destroy the abnormal or foreign material or make it harmless; and most hormones, which regulate various processes. Cells also change fatty acids and glucose to stored energy, each in the form of adipose tissues and glycogen respectively, for later use.

講談社

出典

Carol D. Tamparo *et al.*, *Diseases of the Human Body fourth edition*, F. A. Davis Company (2005)
    [p.14, 15, 135, 136, 153, 154, 209, 210, 213, 214, 222, 223, 224, 244, 245, 274, 281, 282, 302, 317, 318, 343, 358, 359]
Steve Parker, *The Human Body Book*, Dorling Kindersley (2007)
    [p.114, 172, 192]
Mark H. Beers *et al.*, *The Merck Manual of Medical Information Second Home Edition*, Simon & Schuster (2004)
    [p.837, 838]

Preface　まえがき

　今日，管理栄養士を取り巻く状況には変化が見られます．まず，管理栄養士は，医師，看護師，薬剤師など医療系各職種のメンバーで組織される栄養サポートチーム (nutrition support team: NST) の中で，臨床栄養学の視点に基づく治療方法に関する専門家として中心的な役割が期待されるようになりました．さらに，国際栄養士会議 (The International Congress of Dietetics) が日本で初めて開催されるなど (2008年)，日本から国際社会に向け栄養に関する情報を発信する時代となっています．

　本書は，このような医療現場のニーズと養成校におけるカリキュラムに対応して「基礎的な栄養学・医学の専門英語の習得」と「疾病を，英語で医学的・栄養学的に学ぶこと」を意図して作成しました．おもに病院，高齢者福祉施設などで働く管理栄養士 (臨床栄養師) を目指して勉学中の学生およびすでに病院で活躍されている管理栄養士の方々を対象としています．

　食事・栄養管理が必要とされ，日本人に多く見られる疾患から代表的なものを選び，それらを総合的に，効率よく学習するために，以下のように構成しています．

1. 各疾患を医学的観点から食事・栄養管理まで項目別にまとめた英文で理解する．
   [DESCRIPTION] (概説)
   [ETIOLOGY] (病因)
   [SIGNS and SYMPTOMS] (兆候と症状)
   [DIAGNOSIS] (診断)
   [TREATMENT] (治療)
   　1) Medications (薬物療法)
   　2) Dietary management (食事管理)
2. REVIEW QUESTIONSによって内容を確認し，必須英語を習得する．

　専門領域の英語学習はとかく単調になりがちですが，"Let's take a break." で気分転換し，頭の運動をしましょう．

　本書の執筆にあたり，栄養学の専門的立場から貴重なご教示と御助言を賜りました川崎医療福祉大学 中坊幸弘教授ならびに寺本房子教授に心から感謝申し上げます．なお，講談社サイエンティフィク 神尾朋美様には，立案から校正に至るまで詳細に検討していただきました．心からお礼申し上げます．

2013年3月

清水　雅子

J.パトリック バロン

Contents 目次

Unit 1
Gastroenterological System Diseases and Disorders
胃腸管疾患 1
   1. Peptic Ulcer　消化性潰瘍 3
   2. Ulcerative Colitis　潰瘍性大腸炎 7
   3. Cirrhosis　肝硬変 11
   4. Chronic Pancreatitis　慢性膵炎 15

Unit 2
Skeletal System Diseases and Disorders
骨格系疾患 20
   1. Osteoporosis　骨粗鬆症 23

Unit 3
Cardiovascular System Diseases and Disorders
心臓血管系疾患 28
   1. Arteriosclerosis　動脈硬化症 30
   2. Hypertension　高血圧症 34

Unit 4
Nervous System Diseases and Disorders
神経系の疾患 38
   1. Cerebrovascular Accident（Stroke）　脳血管障害（脳卒中） 40
   2. Parkinson Disease　パーキンソン病 45

Unit 5
Respiratory System Diseases and Disorders
呼吸器系疾患 49
   1. Chronic Obstructive Pulmonary Disease　慢性閉塞性肺疾患 51

Unit 6
Urinary System Diseases and Disorders
泌尿器系疾患 55

1. End-stage Renal Diseases (Chronic Renal Failure/Chronic Kidney Disease)
   末期腎疾患（慢性腎不全） 57
2. Nephrotic Syndrome　ネフローゼ症候群 62

Unit 7
Immune-related Diseases and Disorders
免疫系の疾患 66

1. Food Allergy　食物アレルギー 68

Unit 8
Metabolic Diseases and Disorders
代謝疾患 74

1. Dyslipidemia　脂質異常症 76
2. Diabetes Mellitus　糖尿病 80

Unit 9
Nutritional Diseases and Disorders
栄養疾患 87

1. Protein-energy Malnutrition　たんぱく質・エネルギー栄養障害 88
2. Dysphagia (Swallowing Disorder)　嚥下障害 94

Unit 10
Psychogenic Diseases and Disorders
心因性疾患 100

1. Anorexia Nervosa　神経性食欲不振症 102
2. Bulimia Nervosa　神経性大食症 106

Appendix 1　Biochemical Tests of Blood/Urinalysis
血液生化学検査・尿検査 111
Appendix 2　The Names of Diseases and Disorders　疾患の名称 112

Unit 1: Gastroenterological System Diseases and Disorders
胃腸管疾患

Introduction to the Gastroenterological System

What is the gastroenterological system?

The Gastroenterological (digestive) system consists of a long passageway, extending from the mouth to the anus, known as the alimentary canal or digestive tract, and associated organs, including the liver, gallbladder, and pancreas. Along its course, food is broken down and nutrients extracted, while waste materials are passed on.

How does the gastroenterological organs work?

After being eaten, or ingested, food embarks on a journey. It can

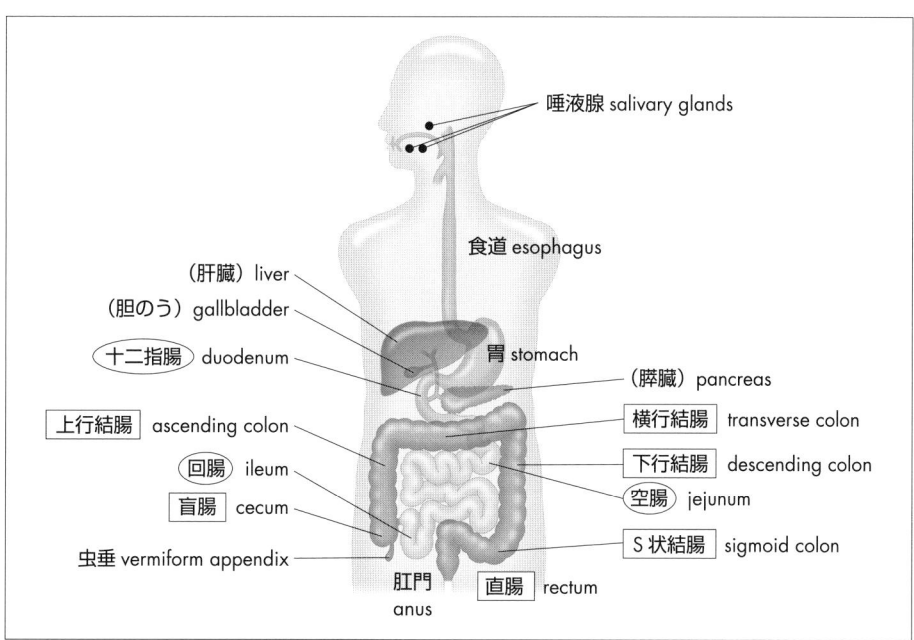

Figure 1 The gastroenterological system（胃腸管）
◯ 小腸 small intestine, ▭ 大腸 large intestine, （ ） 付属消化器官 accessary digestive organs

take up to 24 hours to cover a distance of 30 ft (9 m), through various muscular tubes and chambers. The process begins at the mouth, where food is initially crushed and ground by the teeth during chewing. The resulting ball, or bolus, of food continues down the throat (pharynx), then travels through the food tube (esophagus) to the stomach, small intestine, large intestine, and anus. In the small intestine, chemical digestion breaks down food into molecules small enough to be absorbed into the bloodstream. What cannot be digested is compacted as feces in the large intestine and eliminated as stool through the anus. Food travels the system by a process of muscular contraction called peristalsis.

In addition to the digestive tract, the gastroenterological system includes several glands: the sputum-creating salivary glands; the pancreas, which produces powerful digestive juices; and the body's major nutrient processor, the liver.

1. Peptic Ulcer 消化性潰瘍

　消化性潰瘍は，胃・十二指腸潰瘍の一般的総称である．胃酸やペプシン分泌が強力に促進され，胃壁や腸壁の防御機構である粘膜が侵され，限局性の病変が起きた状態をいう．食道下部，空腸にも発症するが，好発部位は胃の小弯部，幽門部，十二指腸の始まりの部分である．主要な原因はヘリコバクターピロリ菌の感染とアスピリン，非ステロイド薬などの薬剤であるが，ストレス，アルコール，喫煙なども影響があると考えられている．潰瘍は，治癒と再発を繰り返し，慢性化する傾向が強く，痛み，胸やけ，出血，穿孔，便通障害などの症状を起こす．日本では欧米と逆に十二指腸潰瘍よりも胃潰瘍が多くみられる．X線，内視鏡による検査で発見され，薬物療法と緩やかな食事療法がなされる．

KEY WORDS

Select the Japanese term most appropriate for each English term.
1. duodenal ulcer　2. erosion　3. gastric ulcer　4. heartburn
5. irritant　6. mucosa　7. nausea　8. peptic ulcer　9. stomach acid
10. vomiting
a. 胃酸　b. 嘔吐　c. 胃潰瘍　d. 十二指腸潰瘍　e. 消化性潰瘍　f. 刺激物
g. 粘膜　h. 吐き気　i. 胸やけ　j. びらん

[DESCRIPTION]

　A peptic ulcer is a round or oval sore where a small area of the gastric or duodenal mucosa has been eaten by gastric acid and digestive juices. Once the defensive mechanism of the mucosa is broken, peptic ulcer will appear and the stomach and the duodenum begin digesting themselves through the effect of its strong acid and pepsin. As the result, depression or a hole is sometimes made with varied depth into its wall.

[ETIOLOGY]

　The three major causes of peptic ulcers are infection with *Helicobactor pylori*, use of nonsteroidal anti-inflammatory drugs

Helicobactor pylori：学名はイタリック体で表現する．

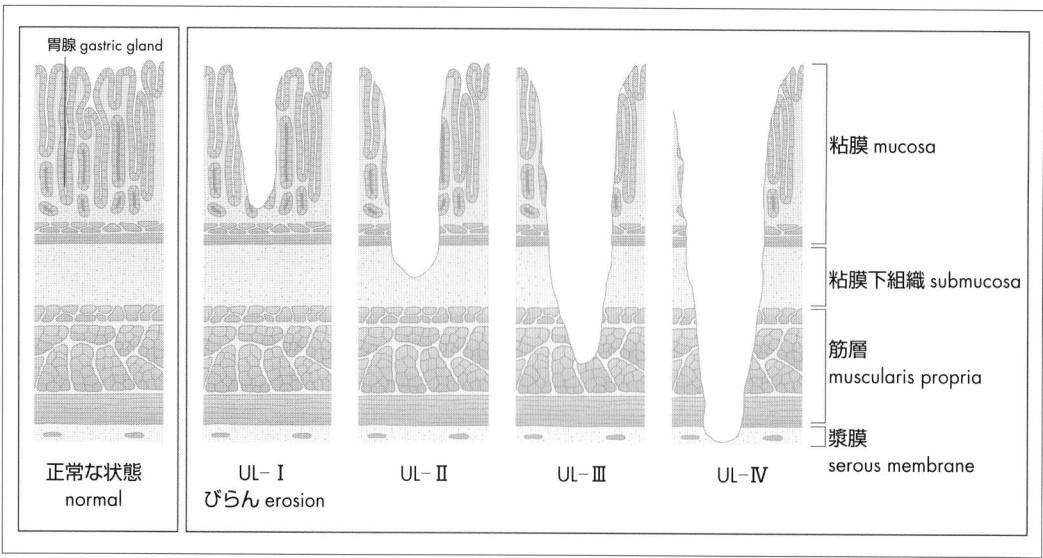

Figure 2 Development of gastric ulcer（胃潰瘍の発生メカニズム）

UL: ulcer. UL-I: erosion (shallow ulcer only limited to the mucosa with no mucosal penetration), UL-II: ulcer that injures the submucosa, UL-III: deep ulcer that reaches the muscular layer, UL-IV: perforating ulcer extending through the wall

(NSAIDs), and pathologic hypersecretion disorders. Just how ulcers develop is not entirely clear, but the process is believed to be related to increased gastric acid production and/or to factors that impair mucosal barrier protection.

[SIGNS and SYMPTOMS]

Persistent "heartburn" and indigestion are the classic symptoms. Gastrointestinal (GI) bleeding, nausea, vomiting, and weight loss can also occur. Chronic, periodic heartburn may radiate into the back region. Often, there is a peculiar sensation of hot water bubbling in the back of the throat. The symptoms of both gastric and duodenal ulcers appear about 2 hours after eating or after consuming fluids containing orange juice, caffeine, alcohol, or aspirin.

[DIAGNOSIS]

Diagnosis is confirmed by esophagogastroduodenoscopy, barium swallow, or a series of x-ray imaging of a small bowel. Laboratory analysis to detect minute quantities of blood, or occult blood in stool, serologic testing to determine clinical signs of infection, studies of

NSAIDs：非ステロイド抗炎症薬．　stool：類語 feces（複数），excrement（排泄物）．

gastric secretions that show hyperchlorhydria, and a carbon 13 (^{13}C) urea breath test results can reflect activity of *H. pylori*.

[TREATMENT]

1) Medication

It is recommended that every person with an ulcer is treated with some of the following drugs.

* Antacids (bicarbonate)
* Acid-reducing drugs; Histamine-2 (H2) blockers
* Proton pump inhibitors
* Miscellaneous drugs

2) Dietary management

Sufficient intakes of nutrients can be more helpful rather than a strictly restricted diet. However, if the patient vomits what he/she ate or discharges blood, they should be told not to drink alcohol and not to eat too much. In addition, such irritants as alcohol, coffee, hot spices, or some other favorite spicy foods are better eliminated.

Small but frequent food intake is desirable for patients but hunger for hours is not good. Stress reduction and non-smoking are also important as risk factors of peptic ulcer.

urea breath test：尿素呼気試験（ピロリ菌の検査法）． small but frequent food intake：少量頻回食（1日3回食を，1日数回に分けて少量にして食べる）．

Let's take a break.

胃腸管の病気のひとつ，消化性潰瘍の項が終わりました．それでは，ちょっとひと休み．なぞなぞ(何ぞ何ぞ)遊びをしましょう．

問：How is that he's troubled with dyspepsia?
答：He tried to spell it.
問：どうして彼は消化不良で悩んでいるの？
答：そのつづりがわからなくて．

日本語に直すと英語のおもしろさは消えてしまいますが，-pepsia は「消化性の」という意味，dys- は「不良」「悪い」などの意味ですから，dyspepsia は消化不良です．でも，彼が悩んでいるのは消化不良ではなくて「つづりがわからない」と言う訳です．spell には「呪文・まじないでしばる」という意味もありますが，深入りしないのが賢明...

REVIEW QUESTIONS

I Select the correct definition for each term.
1. mucosa 2. *Helicobactor pylori* 3. peptic ulcer 4. irritant
5. erosion
   a) A lesion in the mucosa of the digestive tube, typically in the stomach or duodenum, caused by the action of pepsin and stomach acid
   b) A bacterial species that produces urease and is associated with several gastroduodenal diseases
   c) Epithelial tissue that secretes mucus and that lines many body cavities and tubular organs including the gut and respiratory passages
   d) The gradual destruction of tissue by physical or chemical action
   e) A substance that causes light inflammation or corporal discomfort

II Write the appropriate term on the line.
1. A peptic ulcer is a round or _____ of the mucosa of the stomach or duodenum.
2. A peptic ulcer is a condition where the mucous membrane of the _____ or duodenum has been eaten away by stomach acid and _____ juices.
3. The most common causes of peptic ulcer are infection with _____ and use of certain drugs.
4. Persistent _____ and indigestion are classic symptoms of peptic ulcer.
5. _____ may be good for patients but hunger for hours is not good.

III Write T for true, F for false on the line.
1. ____ A peptic ulcer is a lesion, typically in the stomach, eaten away by the stomach acid and pepsin.
2. ____ One of the most common causes identified so far of peptic ulcer is infection with *Helicobactor pylori*.
3. ____ The symptoms of peptic ulcers appear about 6 hours after eating or drinking stimulants, such as coffee, alcohol, or taking aspirin.
4. ____ A strictly restricted diet is recommended to a person with a peptic ulcer.
5. ____ Small but frequent food intake with many kinds of food is good for the patient and hunger for some hours is also good.

2. Ulcerative Colitis　潰瘍性大腸炎

　潰瘍性大腸炎は，大腸の粘膜に炎症を生じ，潰瘍を形成する慢性疾患である．通常，直腸，S状結腸から始まり，大腸の一部，あるいは全体に広がり，激しい腹痛，発熱，出血性下痢を伴う再発性の疾患である．原因は不明だが，遺伝と異物に対する腸の過剰反応とされている．
　治療は，抗炎症の症状を抑える目的で薬剤が中心となるが，食事療法では，炎症のある粘膜を傷つけないように生野菜や果物を避ける．また，乳製品を避けることで症状が軽減することもある．

KEY WORDS
Select the Japanese term most appropriate for each English term.
1. anemia　2. colon　3. dairy product　4. dehydration　5. diet
6. exacerbation　7. foreign body　8. inflammation　9. remission
10. sigmoidoscopy
a. 乳製品　b. 炎症　c. 脱水　d. 異物　e. S状結腸鏡検査法　f. 寛解
g. 結腸　h. 貧血　i. 規定食　j. 増悪

[DESCRIPTION]

　Ulcerative colitis is a chronic inflammation and ulceration of the colon, often beginning in the rectum or sigmoid colon and extending upward into the entire colon. The inflammation involves only the mucosal lining of the colon, which exhibits erythema and numerous hemorrhagic ulcerations.

[ETIOLOGY]

　The etiology of ulcerative colitis is similar to that as Crohn disease. Researchers believe that the body's defenses may be operating against some substance in the body, perhaps even the digestive tract, which are recognized as autoimmune. These foreign bodies or antigens may stimulate the body's defenses to produce an inflammation.

[SIGNS and SYMPTOMS]

　The classic symptom is recurrent bloody diarrhea, often containing

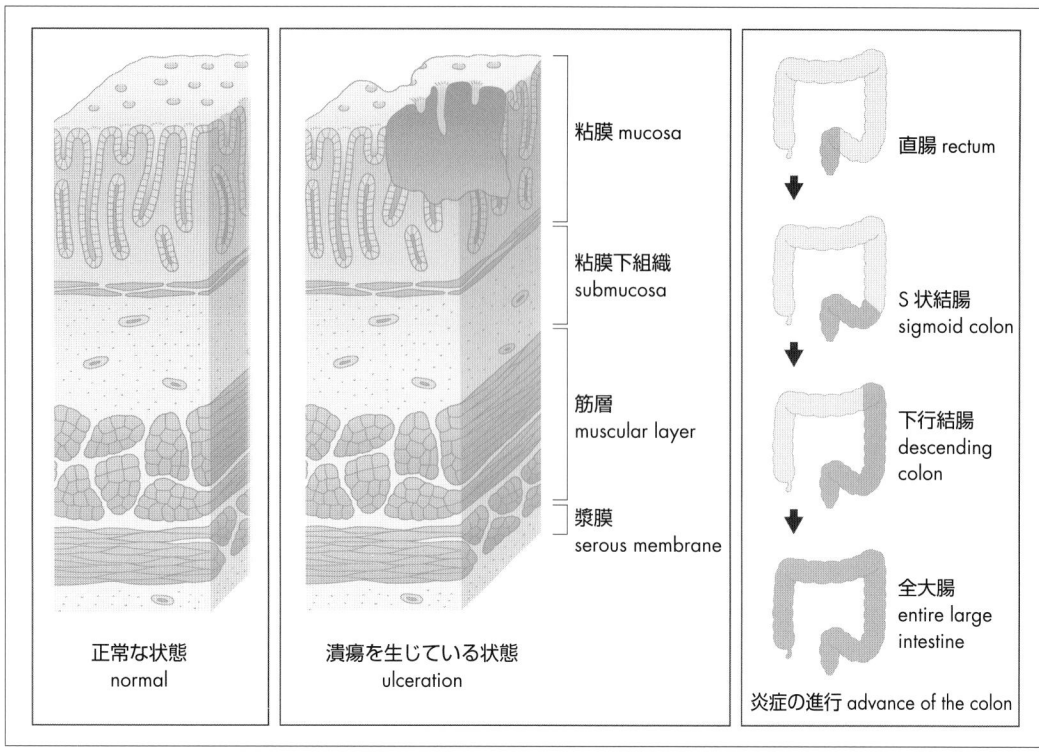

Figure 3　Development of ulceration of the colon（潰瘍性大腸炎の発生メカニズム）

pus and mucus, accompanied by abdominal sensation and severe urgency to move for bowels. Other symptoms may include fever, weight loss, and signs of dehydration. There is a tendency toward periodic exacerbation or improvement of symptoms.

[DIAGNOSIS]

The disease is diagnosed by the characteristics of the inflammatory process. Sigmoidoscopy may reveal the mucosal lining to be friable with thick inflammatory exudates. Colonoscopy may be necessary to determine the extent of the disease, and biopsy may be performed to determine the histologic status.

[TREATMENT]

1) Medication

The treatment program generally includes measures to suppress the inflammatory response and control symptoms. The main medicines are:

＊Sulfasalazine

* Sulfapyridine
* 5-ASA (5-aminosalicylic acid)
* Corticosteroids

2) Dietary management

Iron supplements may offset anemia caused by ongoing blood loss in the stool. Raw fruits and vegetables should be avoided to reduce injury to the inflamed lining of the large intestine. A diet free of dairy products may decrease symptoms and is worth trying but need not be continued if no benefit is noted.

Let's take a break.

あれ？ peptic ulcerにも ulcerative colitisにも ulcerがあるさー？ 冗談はさておき（"Joking aside."），peptic ulcerは gastroduodenal ulcer（胃十二指腸潰瘍）とも言います．ここで専門用語の構成に触れておきましょう．語を分析すると，

* gastro-(胃)＋duoden-(12)＝[du-(2)＋dec-(10)]＋ulcer（ただれ・痛み）
* ulcer＋-ative(-の)／colo-(結腸＋-it is（痛み）

（解剖学用語のラテン語は形容詞が名詞の後ろに位置する．）

となります．通常，専門用語は，接頭辞＋連結（形語根＋接尾辞から構成されています（ただし，この2語には接頭辞がありません）．

さて，このギリシャ語の由来のgastro-は，解剖学・病名・症状・検査・手術用語... と数多くの多彩な用語を作ります．また，gastro-は一般語にも見られ，例えば，gastronomer（食通）（フランス語でgourme：グルメ）．この英語の本来の意味はgastro-＋nom（nomos＝law），つまり，「胃を（規則によって）管理する人」であり，nomosには味や香りだけでなく，栄養学的事実，調理法，食物の知識，盛り付けなどが含まれています．

そして管理栄養士が患者のために食通になるには，特に身体における食物摂取についての知識が，そのためには身体の仕組みと働きと病気の理解が必要とされることは言うまでもありません．

REVIEW QUESTIONS

I Select the correct definition for each term.
  1. chronic   2. colon   3. exudates   4. foreign body   5. erythema
   a) State of lasting for a long time and being difficult to cure
   b) A mass of cells and fluid that has seeped out of blood vessels or organ
   c) An object or piece of extraneous matter that has entered the body by accident
   d) Superficial reddening of the skin, usually in patches
   e) The main part of the large intestine, which passes from the cecum to the rectum

II Write the appropriate term on the line.
  1. Ulcerative colitis is a chronic _____ and ulceration of the _____.
  2. The typical symptom is recurrent bloody _____ with abdominal pain and urgent movement of bowels.
  3. There is a tendency toward periodic _____ and improvement of symptoms.
  4. The disease is diagnosed by the characteristics of the inflammatory process by means of sigmoidoscopy, _____ and a biopsy.
  5. A diet _____ of dairy products may decrease symptoms.

III Write T for true, F for false on the line.
  1.____ Ulcerative colitis is acute inflammation, often of the entire colon.
  2.____ Ulcerative colitis may be produced by roundworm that induces injuries in the body.
  3.____ Bloody diarrhea does not often occur but abdominal pain often occurs simultaneously.
  4.____ Colonoscopy may reveal the mucosal lining to be crumbled with thick inflammatory exudates.
  5.____ Raw fruits and cooked vegetables need not to be eliminated to reduce injury to the inflamed lining of the large intestine.

3. Cirrhosis 肝硬変

慢性肝疾患(ウイルス性肝炎,アルコール性肝障害,原発性胆汁性肝硬変,原発性硬化性胆管炎, ヘモクロマトーシス, 自己免疫性肝炎, ウィルソン病など)が進行し,肝機能が低下,たんぱく質合成ができず,肝不全となり,しばしば肝細胞がんに至る不可逆的疾患である.日本における肝硬変の病因は,C型肝炎ウイルス(約60％)が最も高く,次いで,アルコール(約26％),B型肝炎ウイルス(約12％)である.慢性化すると,門脈周辺の繊維化,消化管から肝臓への血流が阻止され,血液は直接心臓へと流れる.静脈瘤のために血管破裂が起きる.腹水による腹部の拡張(膨満),さまざまな栄養代謝障害,たんぱく質・栄養エネルギー障害を起こす.

KEY WORDS

Select the Japanese term most appropriate for each English term.
1. biosynthesis   2. cirrhosis   3. enzyme   4. fatigability   5. hepatic
6. jaundice   7. malnutrition   8. metabolism   9. protein   10. virus
a. たんぱく質   b. 代謝   c. 栄養障害   d. 疲労性   e. ウイルス   g. 生合成
h. 黄疸   i. 肝硬変   j. 肝臓の   k. 酵素

[DESCRIPTION]

Cirrhosis is a chronic, irreversible, degenerative disease of the liver characterized by the replacement of normal liver cells with fibrous scar tissue and other alterations in liver structure. The hepatic cells become necrotic, causing a change in the liver structure that impairs the flow of blood and lymph resulting in hepatic insufficiency.

[ETIOLOGY]

Cirrhosis has a diverse set of etiologies. The most common cirrhosis is portal, nutritional or alcoholic cirrhosis. Other forms of cirrhosis, classified by their pathogenesis, include biliary cirrhosis, or cholestasis, postnecrotic cirrhosis resulting from hepatitis, pigment cirrhosis, and cardiac cirrhosis. Cirrhosis also may be idiopathic in origin. It is more common in men than in women.

In Japan, cirrhosis is most commonly caused by hepatitis C virus (60%), hepatitis B virus (12%), and alcohol (26%).

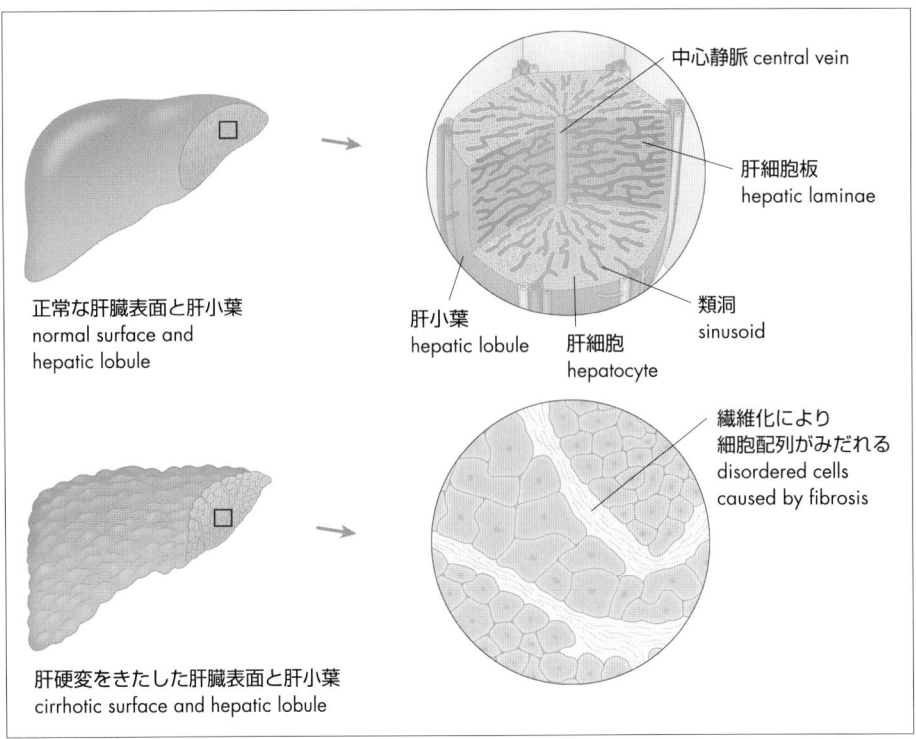

Figure 4 Cirrhosis（肝硬変）

[SIGNS and SYMPTOMS]

The person may be asymptomatic for a prolonged period, or symptoms may be vague or unspecific. Symptoms may include nausea, vomiting, anorexia, dull abdominal ache, weakness, fatigability, weight loss, pruritus, peripheral neuritis, bleeding tendencies, edema of the legs and jaundice.

[DIAGNOSIS]

Plain abdominal x-ray films may show an enlarged liver. A liver scan and biopsy are essential for diagnosis. Laboratory findings may reveal anemia, folate deficiency, blood loss, and rupturing of red blood cells with the resulting release of hemoglobin into the plasma, a process called hemolysis. Liver enzymes (alanine aminotrasferase [ALT] and aspartate aminotransferase [AST]) are assayed to check for elevated enzyme levels. The bilirubin level will also be increased.

[TREATMENT]

1) Medication

Antibiotics will be prescribed for infections, and various medications can reduce itching. Laxatives decrease the risk of constipation, but their role in preventing encephalopathy is limited. Treatment for hepatitis-related cirrhosis involves medications used to treat the different types of hepatitis, such as interferon for viral hepatitis and corticosteroids for autoimmune hepatitis.

2) Dietary management

A healthy balanced diet is encouraged, as cirrhosis is an energy-consuming condition. However, the standard nutritional level shown in the table 2 must be maintained in the dietary management.

The idea of small but frequent food intake may be introduced in order to eliminate sensation of hunger, especially early in the morning. Late evening snack (LES) before going to bed is also recommended.

Table 1 Nutritional metabolic disorder caused by cirrhosis (肝硬変の栄養代謝障害)

energy metabolic disorder	energy hypermetabolism
carbohydrate metabolic disorder	insulin resistance, hyperinsulinemia, hyperglucagonemia, glycogen storage disorder
dyslipidemia	lipolytic acceralation, fatty acid oxidation
protein–amino acid metabolic disorder	protein biosynthesis, protein degradation, protein intolerance, decreasing of Fischer ratio

Table 2 Nutritional standard level for patients with cirrhosis (肝硬変患者の栄養基準)

energy requirement	25–35 kcal/kg (abnormal glucose torelance: 25–30 kcal/kg/day)
protein*	1.0–1.5 g/kg/day (protein intolerance: 0.5–0.7 g/kg/day+enteral feeding)
fat	energy ratio 20–25%
salt	8–9 g/day (ascites/edema 5–7 g/day)

* Granulated BCAA (branched-chain amino acid) may be administered for the patient who has the result of laboratory test; less than 3.5 g/dL (low albumin), less than 1.8 (Fischer ratio), less than 3.0 (BTR: molar ratio of total BCAA to tyrosine).

REVIEW QUESTIONS

I Select the correct definition for each term.
   1. protein   2. malnutrition   3. ascites   4. cirrhosis   5. metabolism
   a) A serious, often fatal disease of the liver caused especially by too much alcohol, but more often by hepatitis C virus in Japan
   b) Any substances that consists of large molecules composed of one or more long chains of amino acids
   c) The chemical processes that occur within a living organism in order to maintain life
   d) A poor condition of health caused by a lack of food or lack of the right type of food
   e) The accumulation of fluid in the peritoneal cavity, causing abdominal swelling

II Write the appropriate term on the line.
   1. Symptoms of cirrhosis include nausea, anorexia, dull abdominal ache, fatigability, edema, _____, etc.
   2. Cirrhosis is characterized by the replacement of normal _____ cells with _____ tissue.
   3. In Japan, cirrhosis is most commonly caused by _____.
   4. Treatment for hepatitis-related cirrhosis involves medications, such as _____ and corticosteroids.
   5. A healthy balanced diet is encouraged, as cirrhosis change into _____ condition.

III Write T for true, F for false on the line.
   1. ____ Cirrhosis is a reversible disease of the liver characterized by proliferation of cells, inflammation, and fibrous thickening.
   2. ____ Cirrhosis in Japan is typically caused by drinking too much alcohol.
   3. ____ A person with cirrhosis sometimes shows no symptoms.
   4. ____ Laboratory tests as well as abdominal x-ray film, liver scan and biopsy are essential for diagnosis.
   5. ____ The idea of small but frequent food intake is introduced to remove the sensation of hunger early in the morning.

4. Chronic Pancreatitis　慢性膵炎

　慢性膵炎の病因は大部分がアルコール過飲であり，その他は膵管閉塞，先天的要因などであるが，原因不明も多い．膵臓の炎症が長期間続き，機能低下を生じる再発性の慢性疾患であり，代償期と非代償期に分かれ，さらに代償期は間欠期と急性再燃期に分類される．代償期には炎症および腹部・背部の疼痛，急性再燃期には上腹部の持続的疝痛，悪心，嘔吐，非代償期には腹部痛は軽減し，消化酵素の分泌低下によって食物の消化吸収障害が起きる，また，高血糖，低血糖の症状を示す．

　食事療法としては，絶飲食から常食まで代償期，急性再燃期，非代償期における症状に合わせた食事形態で管理する．

KEY WORDS

Select the Japanese term most appropriate for each English term.
1. alcoholism　2. computed tomography (CT)　3. enteral nutrition
4. flare-ups　5. general diet　6. hyperglycemia　7. irreversible
8. nothing by mouth　9. parenteral hyperalimentation
10. rice gruel diet
a. 粥食　b. 常食　c. 再燃(再発)　d. 高血糖　e. 絶飲食
f. 非経腸栄養[法]　g. 経腸栄養[法]　h. アルコール中毒　i. 不可逆的
j. コンピュータ断層撮影法

[DESCRIPTION]

　Chronic pancreatitis is persistent inflammation of the pancreas that results in progressive and irreversible worsening of its structure and function. With necrosis of the parenchyma, membranes of the cells begin to exfoliate, and finally fibrosis develops. As a result, the function of the pancreas starts deteriorating.

[ETIOLOGY]

　The causes of this autodigestive process in pancreatitis are not well understood, although a number of conditions are known to lead to the disease. Chief among these, alcoholism is (mostly in men) the main etiologic and biliary tract disease (more common in women). Other conditions include gallstones, abdominal trauma, viral infections,

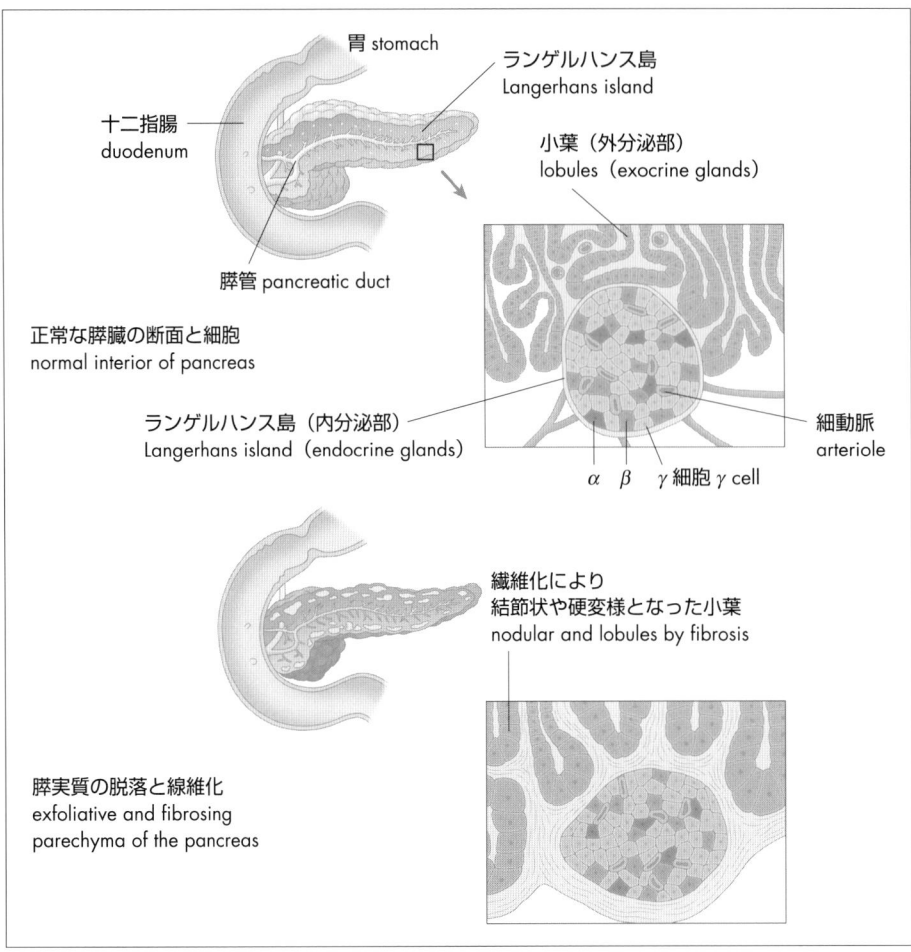

Figure 5　Chronic pancreatitis（慢性膵炎）

drug reactions, systemic immunologic disorders, pancreatic cancer, or complications from a duodenal ulcer.

[SIGNS and SYMPTOMS]

Symptoms with chronic pancreatitis generally fall into two types, with flare-ups and no-flare-ups. During flare-ups, a person has abdominal and back pain that varies in intensity with inflammation by digestive enzymes after eating. However, conditions in the acute flare-ups are similar to those of acute pancreatitis. If there are no-flare-ups, abdominal pain diminishes. The chief symptoms are disorders of digestion and absorption caused by the decline of the digestive enzymes, and hyperglycemia as well as hypoglycemia due to the declining function of insulin and glucagon secretions.

[DIAGNOSIS]

In addition to clinical symptoms, diagnostic imaging, computed tomography (CT) scans, endoscopic retrograde cholangiopancreatography (ERCP) are performed, and blood biochemistry are usually tested. The value of serum amylase or lipase is normally high, but when the flare-ups come, these tend to be even higher.

[TREATMENT]

1) Medication

Medical treatment is largely symptomatic. Analgesic drugs, intravenous administration of fluids, and fasting with parenteral hyperalimentation to maintain normal growth and development and to provide for needed tissue repair may be necessary.

2) Dietary management

(1) During an acute flare-up, avoiding all food and drink except intravenous drip is necessary. With a recovery from pain, the patient gradually starts oral intake, and then, moves to the liquid food such as rice gruel (*omoyu*) or starch gruel (*kuzuyu*) before moving to

endoscopic retrograde cholangiopancreatography（ERCP）：内視鏡的逆行性胆管膵管造影［法］　analgesic drug：鎮痛薬　parenteral hyperalimentation：非経口的栄養療法．栄養には十分なアミノ酸，グルコース，脂肪酸，電解質，ビタミン，ミネラルを含む．

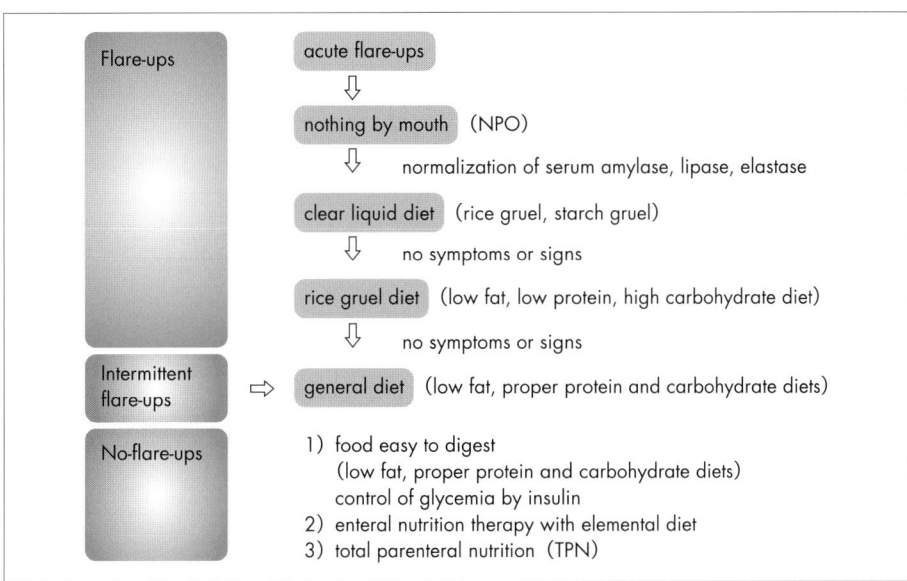

Figure 6　Dietary management for chronic pancreatitis（慢性膵炎の栄養管理）

general diet. Lipid (taken orally) are also added little by little, according to the person's condition.

(2) In case of intermittent flare-ups, the general therapeutic diet basically limits the lipid quantity (30–40 g). Deep fried food should be avoided because of their levels of enough oils and fats. Protein does not need to be restricted (1.0–1.2 g/kg/day) for standard body weight. Carbohydrates are also taken if there is no glucose tolerance disorder. The patient must avoid drinking caffeine, carbonated drinks, alcohol as well as spices or stimulants.

(3) When there are noflare-ups, restriction of lipid intake is less strict as abdominal pain and inflammation declines. However, digestive and absorptive disorders or fatty stool can appear because external secretion of digestive enzymes declines so that low nutritional status may occur. To prevent these conditions, moderate dosage of digestive enzymes will be helpful.

Though a gruel diet enables easy absorption, high fiber foods should be avoided. Attention should be paid to hyperglycemia or hypoglycemia with low secretion of insulin and glucagon. For hyperglycemia, the diet management is practiced on the basis of the diet therapy for diabetes mellitus, together with the use of insulin.

Let's take a break.

You tell'em, Salad,
　　I'm dressing.
言っておやりよ　サラダさん
　　今，着替えているところ．

　これは，2行で書かれるThe You-Tell-'Em（言っておやりよ）という言葉のごろ合わせ遊びです．この落ち (the point of joke) はdressingです．be dressingは「服を着ているところ」という動詞の進行形．前回のbreakでコメントしたgastronomerはサラダにかけるdressingのほうに通じているのです，よね？

　さて，サラダのa green salad（青野菜）ですが，greenがなぜ青なのだろう？それはさておき，cirrhosis（肝硬変）のcirrho-が黄褐色の意味であるように，医学用語には色彩語がよく含まれています．その話はいずれまた．

REVIEW QUESTIONS

I Select the correct definition for each term.
1. enteral nutrition therapy   2. irreversible   3. intravenous alimentation
4. gruel diet   5. nothing by mouth

   a) Fasting and no liquids intake
   b) A thin liquid food of meal boiled in water
   c) Providing the body with nutrition by intravenous injection
   d) A condition cannot be changed back to what it was before
   e) A kind of alimentation provided by means of a tube inserted into the intestine or gastrointestinal tract

II Write the appropriate term on the line.
1. Chronic pancreatitis is persistent inflammation of the pancreas that results in progressive and _____ deterioration of its structures and functions.
2. Among a number of conditions, alcoholism _____ is the chief etiology.
3. Symptoms of chronic pancreatitis generally fall into two types, those with _____ and no-flare-ups.
4. Fasting with _____ to maintain normal growth and development, and to provide for needed tissue repair, may be necessary.
5. With a recovery from pain, the patient gradually starts oral intake, and then, moves to the liquid food such as rice gruel _____ or starch gruel _____ before taking the general diet.

III Write T for true, F for false on the line.
1. ____ The condition of chronic pancreatitis is able to be turned back to what it was.
2. ____ Among a number of conditions, alcoholism is the chief cause in men, and biliary tract diseases in women.
3. ____ The doctor establishes a diagnoses by use of endoscopy or computed tomography, but not by clinical symptoms.
4. ____ A patient goes on a fast and no drinks (no liquids) during flare-ups.
5. ____ Limitation of lipid intake is more loose in no-flare-ups case.

Skeletal System Diseases and Disorders
骨格系疾患

Introduction to the Skeletal System

What is the skeletal system?

The skeletal system of the human body consists of about 206 bones which make up almost 20% of the body weight. Of the 206 bones, 80 are in the axial skeleton, with 64 in the upper appendicular skeleton and 62 in the lower appendicular skeleton. The axial skeleton consists of the skull, vertebral column (vertebrae and fibrous discs between them), ribs and the sternum.

The bone consists of the compact bone tissue, trabecular bone (also called cancellous or spongy bone) and bone marrow in the medullary space. About two-thirds of the bone matrix is mineral, calcium-phosphates, and carbonate (compact substance), and the rest is almost collagen, the fibrous protein. The outer surface of the bone is covered the periosteum. The end of each bone covered with articular cartilage meets at the site called the joint. The capsule around the joint and a short band of flexible and tough ligaments join two bones. Inside the joint, there is the synovial cavity which secretes synovial fluid.

How does the skeleton work?

The skeleton, a strong and flexible frame of the body, has this following five main functions.

1. Supporting the body and keeping its shape

The skeleton provides a frame to support the muscles and internal organs and the body. The axial skeleton supports the upright postures

---

206：幼児の骨は約270個であるが，成人では融合癒着が生じ約200 〜 206個となる．

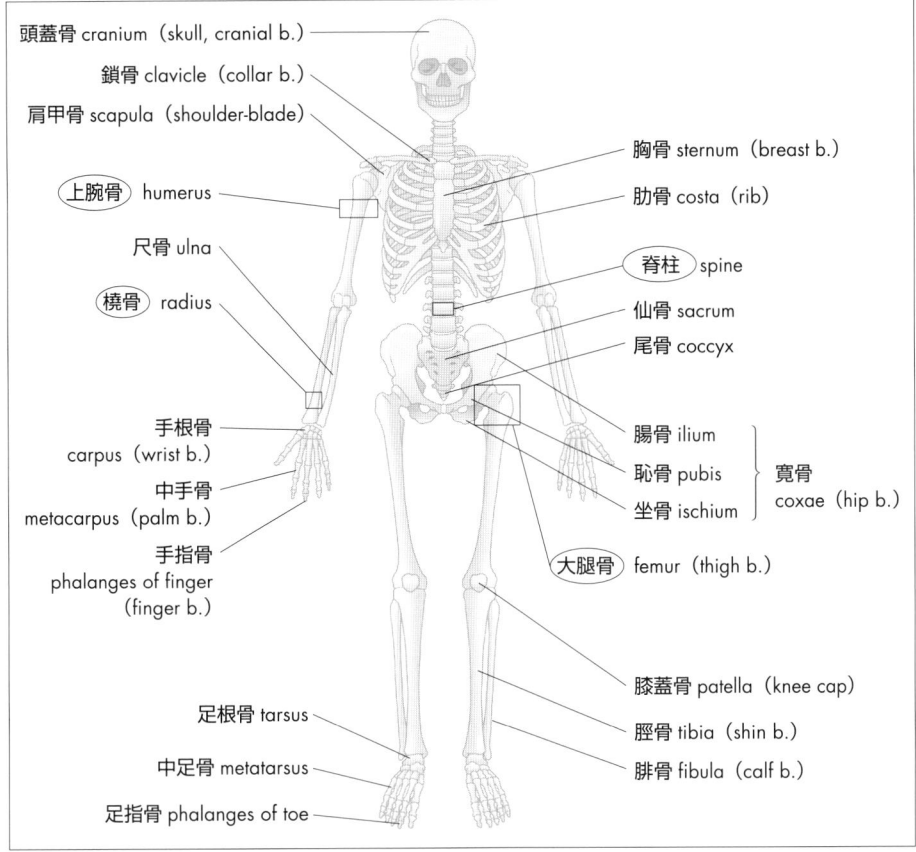

Figure 7　The skeletal system（骨格系）

◯：カルシウムが溶け出しやすく，骨折しやすい部位．　b.：bone

with the help of many ligaments. Mass of bones together with the muscles, ligaments and tendons shape the hands, legs, hips, etc.

2. Protecting important organs

　The skeleton is strong as steel, and surrounds and protects certain vital organs. The skull protects the delicate brain, the ribs and sternum protects the heart and the lungs, and the spinal vertebrae protect the fragile spinal cord.

3. Moving joints

　Joints between the bones make the skeleton able to move or balance with muscles. Many small bones at the joint permit a forward and backward motion from one place to another.

4. Storage of minerals

　Bones are a storage place of minerals, especially calcium which is essential for contraction of the body muscles. Other minerals such as phosphorus, potassium, manganese and others are also preserved in bones.

5. Blood cell production

Blood constitution (red blood cells, white blood cells and platelets) is produced in the soft gelatinous bone marrow in the center of the bone.

1. Osteoporosis　骨粗鬆症

　骨粗鬆症とは，大腿骨，上腕骨，橈骨，脊椎からカルシウムが溶け出し，骨質が減少する全身性代謝疾患をいう．骨量が骨量頂値（最大骨量）の70％未満が骨粗鬆症と診断され，「原発性骨粗鬆症」と「続発性骨粗鬆症」に分類される．特に女性の閉経に伴う「閉経後骨粗鬆症」と加齢による「老人性骨粗鬆症」が前者の90％を占め，後者は内分泌代謝異常や消化管疾患などによるものである．骨粗鬆症は悪化すると骨折を起こしやすくなり，特に足の付け根の骨折は寝たきりを招き認知症になることもある．病気の進行を予防するためには，薬剤投与，長期にわたるカルシウム，ビタミンD，ビタミンKなどを多く摂取する食事療法と，適度の運動を継続する必要がある．また，若いころからバランスのとれた食事，禁煙，適度の飲酒，運動などの予防を意識した生活習慣，食生活が重要である．

KEY WORDS

Select the Japanese term most appropriate for each English term.
1. bone density　2. bone matrix　3. bone scintiscan
4. dual-energy x-ray absorptiometry　5. fracture　6. muscle relaxant
7. peak bone mass　8. postmenopausal　9. vitamin D deficiency
10. μg

a. 筋弛緩剤　b. 骨シンチスキャン　c. 骨密度　d. 骨基質　e. 骨折
f. 骨量頂値　g. マイクログラム　h. 閉経後
i. 二重エネルギーX線吸収測定法　j. ビタミンD欠乏症

[DESCRIPTION]

　Osteoporosis is a metabolic bone disease in which the bone density weakens, and the bone may fracture from even minor injuries. The proportion of bone material to bone matrix is normal, and there usually is no detectable abnormality of bone composition. According to The Japanese Society for Bone and Mineral Research, osteoporosis is diagnosed when 30% of peak bone mass is lost. There are two types of osteoporosis: primary and secondary. The most common form is

The Japanese Society for Bone and Mineral Research：日本骨代謝学会．　peak bone mass：一般的に骨量は20歳から45歳の間に最大となる．　primary and secondary：原発性骨粗鬆症，続発性骨粗鬆症

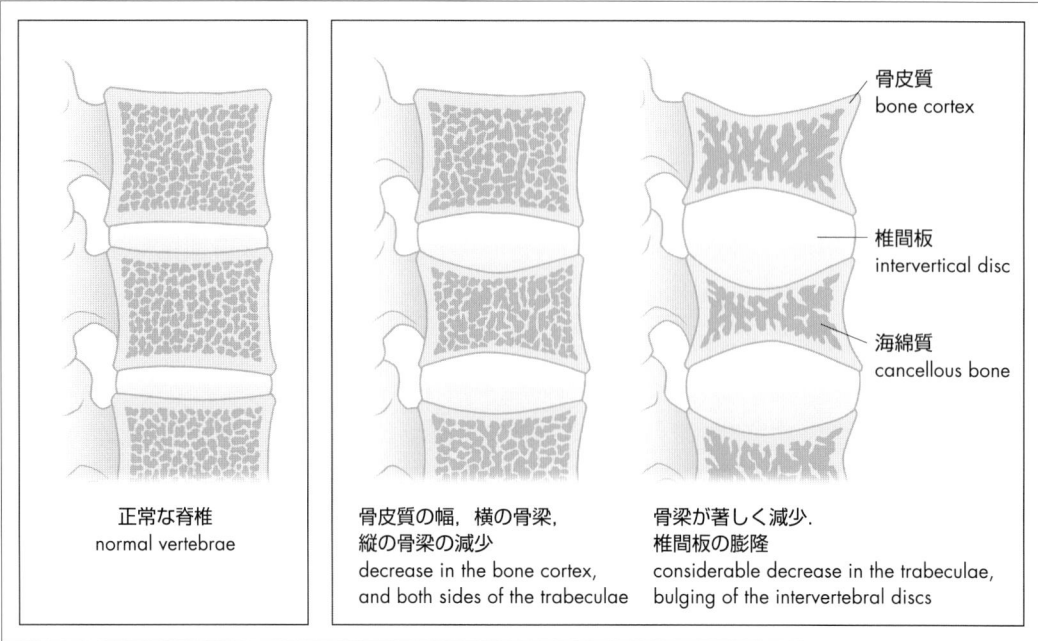

Figure 8　Osteoporosis（骨粗鬆症）

primary osteoporosis which affects women who are past menopause because of lack of estrogens which accelerates bone loss in women. Recently, osteoporosis in young women around 20 years old who go on extreme diets is also becoming a problem.

[ETIOLOGY]

Recent research indicates that heredity plays a role in osteoporosis. Genes influence bone density. In some instances, osteoporosis is a manifestation of another disease, prolonged steroid therapy, alcoholism, lactose intolerance, or hyperthyroidism. Possible contributing factors to osteoporosis include low lifetime intake of calcium, a diet high in protein and fat, a sedentary lifestyle, poor or declining adrenal function, faulty protein metabolism due to estrogen deficiency, vitamin D deficiency, low testosterone levels in men who smoke cigarettes.

[SIGNS and SYMPTOMS]

Symptoms of osteoporosis may go undiscovered until there is a fracture, mostly because the disorder has long been considered a "traumatic" condition. Symptoms will include bone pain, especially in the lower back and in the weight-bearing bones. The vertebrae, hips, and wrists are particularly susceptible to osteoporotic fractures. Patients may notice a loss of height or a humpback.

[DIAGNOSIS]

Recently, a method called dual-energy x-ray absorptiometry (DEXA) to measure bone mineral density at sites especially susceptible to fracture allows physicians to diagnose osteoporosis before any fracture occurs. Blood tests are run to measure levels of phosphorus, alkaline phosphatase, total protein, albumin, and creatinine, and hydroxyproline also may be monitored through urinalysis. A bone scintiscan, bone biopsy, or CT scan may be ordered if more specific diagnostic data are necessary.

[TREATMENT]

1) Medication

The goal is to prevent fracture and control pain. Increased dietary calcium, phosphate supplements, and multivitamins may be prescribed. Bisphosphonates are now the first treatment of choice for both men and women with osteoporosis. Calcium and vitamin D may be provided as supplements to support bone metabolism. Analgesics and muscle relaxants may be needed if pain or muscle spasms are a problem.

2) Exercise

Exercise and walking outside helps minimize osteoporosis by

alkaline phosphatase：アルカリフォスファターゼ．多くのアルカリ性に至適pHをもつ（pH 10前後）正リン酸物エステルを加水分解する酵素の総称．肝・胆道疾患などに高値を示す．

Table 3 Nutritional standards（栄養基準）

calcium (for bone formation)	800 mg/day, calcium-magnesium ratio: 2 : 1
vitamin D (for fast absorption of calcium in the intestine)	700–800 IU* (100 μg/day)
vitamin K	82 μg/day according to dietary reference intake
protein	50 g/day according to the dietary reference intake
salt	10 g/day

* IU : international unit

slowing loss of mineral calcium, but if the bones have become brittle, exercise may need to be modified to prevent injury.

3) Dietary management

As it is impossible to be restored, if the bone matrix is once lost, the treatment aims at preventing the progress of the condition. Keeping dietary intake of calcium, magnesium, vitamin D and K, and protein diets is essential. The standard intakes are shown above.

Let's take a break.

英語には，Knock, knock jokeという広く知られている言葉遊びがあります．そして，そのジョークはパターンが決まっています．

Knock, knock.	とん，とん．
Who's there?	どなたですか？
Lettuce.	レタスです．
Lettuce who?	レタスどなた？
Lettuce in and you'll find out.	入れてくださればわかります．

第1行：ドアをノックする．
第2行：相手の名を尋ねる．
第3行：名前(first name)を答える．
第4行：姓を尋ねる．
第5行：名前にかけたジョークで答える．

この言葉遊びは，アメリカで禁酒法があった時代（1920～1930頃），人々がもぐり酒場のドアをknockして名前や合い言葉を告げたことから始まりました．その後，lettuce＝let usのように，人名以外もしゃれに用いるようになりました．

さて，管理栄養士を目指す方たちには"Knock, and the door will be opened."（新約聖書から）のほうが相応しいかもしれません．

REVIEW QUESTIONS

I Select the correct definition for each term.
1. dual-energy x-ray absorptiometry   2. fracture   3. bone density
4. bone matrix   5. peak bone mass
   a) The amount of mineral content of bone used as an indirect indicator of osteoporosis and fracture risk
   b) The intercellular substance of bone, consisting of collagen fibers, ground substance, and inorganic salts.
   c) An imaging test to measure bone mineral content by passing radiation with two different energies
   d) The average value of a largest amount of bone mineral content in people with between 20 and 40
   e) A crack or break in a hard object or material, typically a bone or cartilage

II Write the appropriate term on the line.
1. The most common form of _____ osteoporosis affects women who are past _____ because of lack of estrogen.
2. Bones become brittle, porous, and vulnerable to fracture due to the decreased _____ and _____ in bones.
3. The proportion of bone material to _____ is normal, however, there usually is no detectable abnormality of bone composition.
4. Symptoms of osteoporosis may go undiscovered until there is a presenting _____.
5. A tool called _____ to measure bone mineral density allows diagnosis of osteoporosis before any fracture occurs.

III Write T for true, F for false on the line.
1. ____ The most common form of primary osteoporosis affects menopausal women because of hormonal unbalance.
2. ____ Only high lifetime intake of calcium is essential for preventing osteoporosis.
3. ____ Symptoms include bone pain, especially in the lower back and in the weight-bearing bones.
4. ____ Medications and exercise are not helpful to prevent fragility of bones because of the irreversible condition of osteoporosis.
5. ____ To prevent the progress of the condition, maintaining intake of calcium, magnesium, vitamin D and K, and protein in diets is essential.

Cardiovascular System Diseases and Disorders
心臓血管系疾患

Introduction to the Cardiovascular System

What is the cardiovascular system?

The cardiovascular (circulatory) system is composed of the heart, blood vessels, and blood. Although the heart is linked to emotions and virtues, such as love and courage, it is basically just a muscular pump. Its regular contractions send blood into tough, elastic tubes, which branch into smaller vessels and convey oxygen-rich blood through the body. The arteries eventually divide into tiny capillaries, which have such thin walls that oxygen, nutrients, minerals, and other substances pass through to surrounding cells and tissues. Waste products flow from the tissues and cells into the blood for

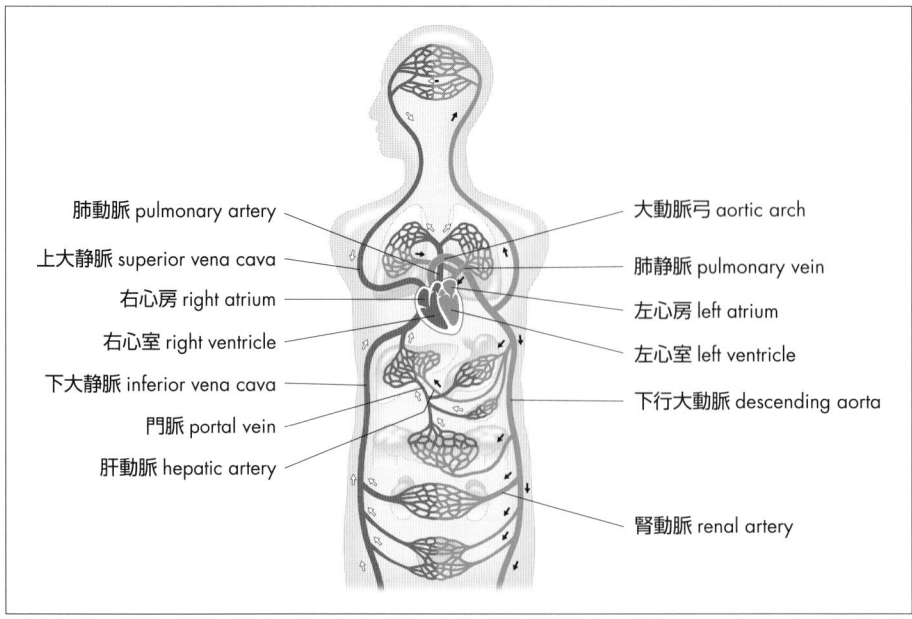

Figure 9　The cardiovascular system（心臓血管系）

disposal. The capillaries join and enlarge to create tubes that eventually become veins, which take blood back to the heart.

How does the cardiovascular system work?

The cardiovascular system is responsible for delivering oxygen and other nutrients to virtually all body cells and removing carbon dioxide and other waste products from them. Like the nervous and lymphatic systems, this complex network extends into every crevice of the body.

Blood is a collection of specialized cells suspended in straw-colored liquid called plasma. Blood delivers oxygen and nutrients to body cells, collects waste, distributes hormones, spreads heat around the body to control temperature, and plays a part in fighting infection and healing injuries.

The heart is a powerful organ about the size of a clenched adult fist. Located just to the left center of the body between the lungs, it operates as a combination of two coordinated pumps that send blood around the body.

1. Arteriosclerosis　動脈硬化症

　心臓から全身に栄養と酸素を運ぶ動脈は，本来，強く弾力性のある血管であるが，主として加齢により徐々に弱く脆くなっていく．加えて，脂質異常，高血圧，肥満，遺伝的素因，喫煙，あるいはストレスなどによって，動脈腔が硬化，肥厚し，病的な動脈硬化が引き起こされる．それはアテローム硬化(粥状)と非アテローム硬化(細動脈およびメンケベルク動脈硬化)に大きく分類されるが，通常，動脈硬化症とは，重大な病状に至るアテローム硬化をさす．特に，状態を悪化させる悪玉コレステロールと呼ばれるコレステロールが長い時間をかけて大・中血管壁に沈着し，粥状のプラークを形成させる．プラークは血栓，塞栓を形成し，脳梗塞，心筋梗塞のような致命的疾患のリスクファクターとなる．このような意味で，最近，日本においてもライフスタイルの改善，内臓型肥満，高血圧，脂質異常症の予防，さらに合併症の予防が国民的課題となっている．

KEY WORDS

Select the Japanese term most appropriate for each English term.
1. aortic aneurysm　2. arterial lumen　3. arteriograms
4. atherosclerosis　5. cerebral thrombosis
6. dietary reference intake　7. dilation　8. obstruction　9. plaque
10. vasodilators
a. 拡張　b. 血管拡張剤　c. 食事摂取基準　d. 動脈内腔　e. 脳血栓
f. 粥状硬化　g. 大動脈瘤　h. 動脈造影　i. プラーク　j. 閉塞

[DESCRIPTION]

　Arteriosclerosis is widespread thickening of the walls of arteries and arterioles, with a resulting loss of elasticity. One type of arteriosclerosis is atherosclerosis, which is a condition characterized by the accumulation of yellowish plaques consisting of cholesterol, lipids, and cellular debris on the inner layers of the walls of large and medium-sized arteries. The vessel walls become thickened, fibrotic, and calcified, and the arterial lumen narrows.

　As a result, the following diseases can occur, especially in men.
* myocardial infarction, angina pectoris (heart)
* cerebral apoplexy: cerebral infarction, cerebral thrombosis (brain)

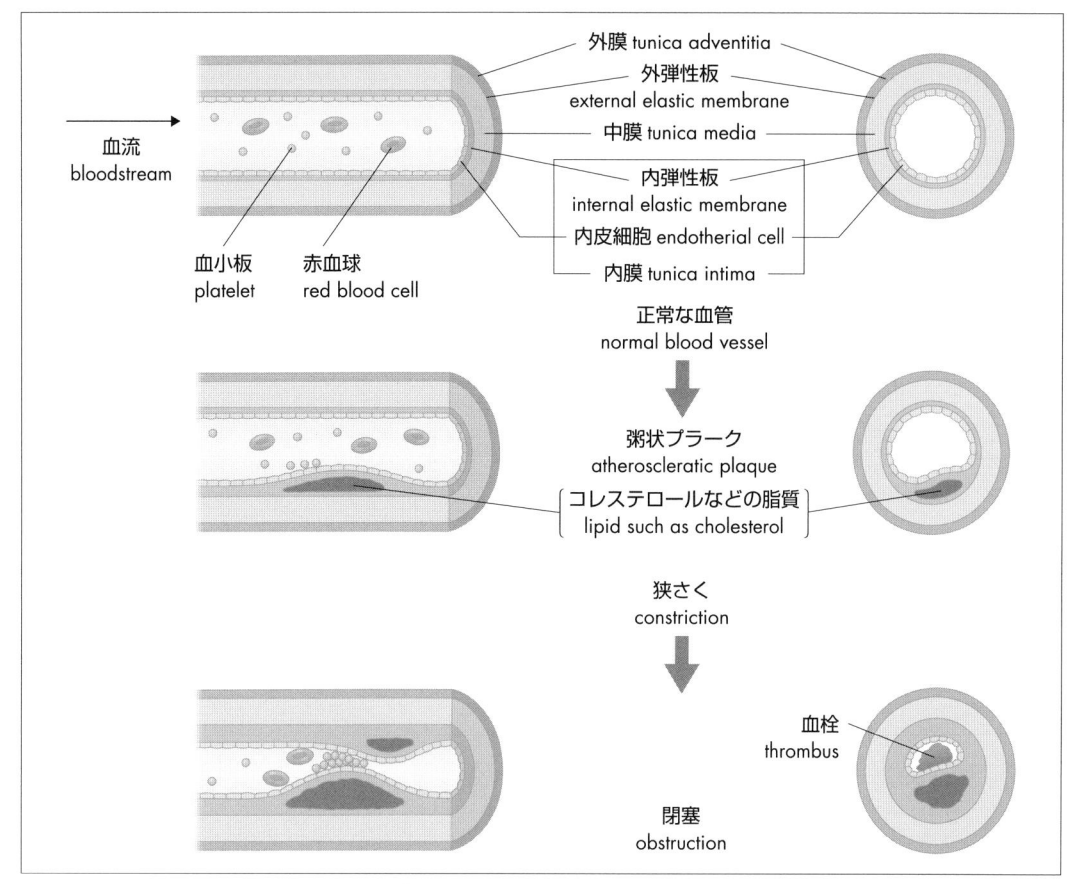

Figure 10 Arteriosclerosis (動脈硬化症)

* arteriosclerosis (foot)
* aortic aneurysm, aortic dissection (large artery)

[ETIOLOGY]

The etiology is unclear, and it is complicated and multifaceted. It may include trauma or the accumulation of lipids due to dietary excesses, faulty carbohydrate metabolism, a sedentary lifestyle, cigarette smoking, stress, or genetic defect. Both pathological changes are seen with aging and are often associated with risk factors such as diabetes mellitus, hypertension, obesity, hyperlipidemia, impaired glucose tolerance, and kidney disorders.

[SIGNS and SYMPTOMS]

The signs and symptoms depend on the blood vessels involved and the extent of blood vessel obstruction. Often the person is asymptomatic. If symptomatic, typical signs and symptoms include intermittent claudication, changes in skin temperature and color, bruits over the involved artery, headache, dizziness, and memory defects. Pain may be present, especially at night, due to sepsis or ischemia. Muscle cramping may occur. The effects of atherosclerosis are gradual stenosis, thrombosis, and subsequent weakening of the blood vessel with dilation.

[DIAGNOSIS]

A diagnosis is often made during routine physical examinations. X-ray films, arteriograms, and blood pressure measurements may be done for diagnosis. Laboratory tests indicate elevated cholesterol, triglyceride, and lipid levels.

[TREATMENT]

The essential treatment for atherosclerosis as one type of arteriosclerosis is lifestyle modification a healthy diet along with physical activity, and abstinence from smoking. Medicines (vasodilators) and medical procedures (surgical removal of a thrombus, together with thromboendarterectomy, and sympathectomy) are also needed.

1) Dietary management

A diet of low unsaturated fats and cholesterol, and vasodilators combined with exercise may be tried. Elimination as well as control of risk factors described above is basic for dietary management. Though clinical dietitians follow dietary reference intakes, they need to take the patients' complications into consideration. The standard of diet control therapy for Japanese with arteriosclerosis is:

a) energy: 25-30 kcal/kg (to keep BMI)
b) cholesterol: less than 200 mg/day
c) animal fat ratio: $P:S=1:2$
d) dietary fiber: more than 10 g/1,000 kcal
e) alcohol: less than 30 g/day
f) sodium chloride (salt): less than 6 g/day

---

thromboendarterectomy：血管内膜切除. P：polyunsaturated fatty acid（多価不飽和脂肪酸）. S：saturated fatty acid（飽和脂肪酸）.

REVIEW QUESTIONS

I Select the correct definition for each term.
  1. thrombosis   2. obstruction   3. plaque   4. infarction
  5. dietary reference intakes
   a) A set of values for the dietary nutrient intakes for the general public and health professionals, used for planning and assessing diets
   b) A condition appearing when the blood supply to an area of tissue is suddenly blocked and the local tissue lacks of oxygen and die
   c) Blockage of flow or movement in a bodily passageway, as blood vessels or intestines
   d) A small, distinct and raised regional fatty deposit on an artery wall in atherosclerosis
   e) A serious condition caused by coagulation or clotting of the blood inside a blood vessel, obstructing vascular flow

II Write the appropriate term on the line.
  1. Atherosclerosis is characterized by the accumulation of _____ of fatty materials on the inner walls of the arteries.
  2. The etiology of arteriosclerosis may include trauma or the accumulation of lipids due to _____ and faulty carbohydrate _____, and so forth.
  3. The effects of atherosclerosis are gradual lumen obstruction, _____, and subsequent weakening of the vessel with dilation.
  4. The essential treatment for atherosclerosis is _____ modification.
  5. Though clinical dietitians follow _____, they need to take the patients' complications into consideration.

III Write T for true, F for false on the line.
  1.____ Arteriosclerosis is local thickening of the walls of large arteries with a resulting decrease of elasticity.
  2.____ Atherosclerosis is deposition of yellowish plaques of cholesterol, lipids on the outer layers of the walls of the arteries.
  3.____ Atherosclerosis is seen with aging and is often associated with diabetes mellitus, hypertension, obesity, hyperlipidemia, etc.
  4.____ The effects of atherosclerosis are acute lumen trauma, thrombosis, and subsequent weakening of the heart.
  5.____ The essential treatments for atherosclerosis are lifestyle changes because medication can be hazardous for patients.

2. Hypertension　高血圧症

　高血圧症とは，心臓から送りだされる血液が血管壁にかかる圧力が高い状態をいう．現在，日本には約4000万人（特に高齢者の60％）が高血圧であると見なされている．高血圧症は病因によって本態性高血圧と2次性高血圧に分類されるが，本態性高血圧が高血圧症の95％を占める．原因は不明であるが，加齢，塩分の多い食事，アルコール，肥満，ストレス，遺伝などに起因して動脈硬化を起こし，血圧が上昇すると考えられる．さらに高血圧は糖尿病や脂質異常症などの合併症を誘発しやすく，また無症状であるために徐々に進行し，放置すると脳梗塞，脳出血のような致命的疾患に至る場合があるので，"silent killer"とも呼ばれている．何よりも食生活を含む生活習慣の改善が必要とされる．

KEY WORDS

Select the Japanese term most appropriate for each English term.
1. auscultation　2. blood pressure　3. constriction of the arteries
4. diastolic pressure　5. electrocardiography　6. Hg　7. idiopathic
8. palpitation　9. systolic pressure　10. tinnitus

a. 拡張期血圧　b. 収縮期血圧　c. 血圧　d. 心電計　e. 水銀　f. 聴診
g. 特発性　g. 動脈狭窄　h. 動悸　i. 耳鳴り

[DESCRIPTION]

　In Japan, hypertension (high blood pressure) has lately drawn considerable attention, because estimated 40,000,000 Japanese people are hypertensive (about 1/3 of the entire Japanese population). What constitutes hypertension may be different for each person and vary with a person's age, gender, and any concomitant disease. It is divided into two types: essential (primary or idiopathic) hypertension and secondary hypertension. Essential hypertension that accounts for 95% of the hypertensive patients is persistently elevated blood pressure without apparent causes. Secondary hypertension develops as the result of various diseases (e.g. renal disease, endocrine tumors, or constriction of the arteries).

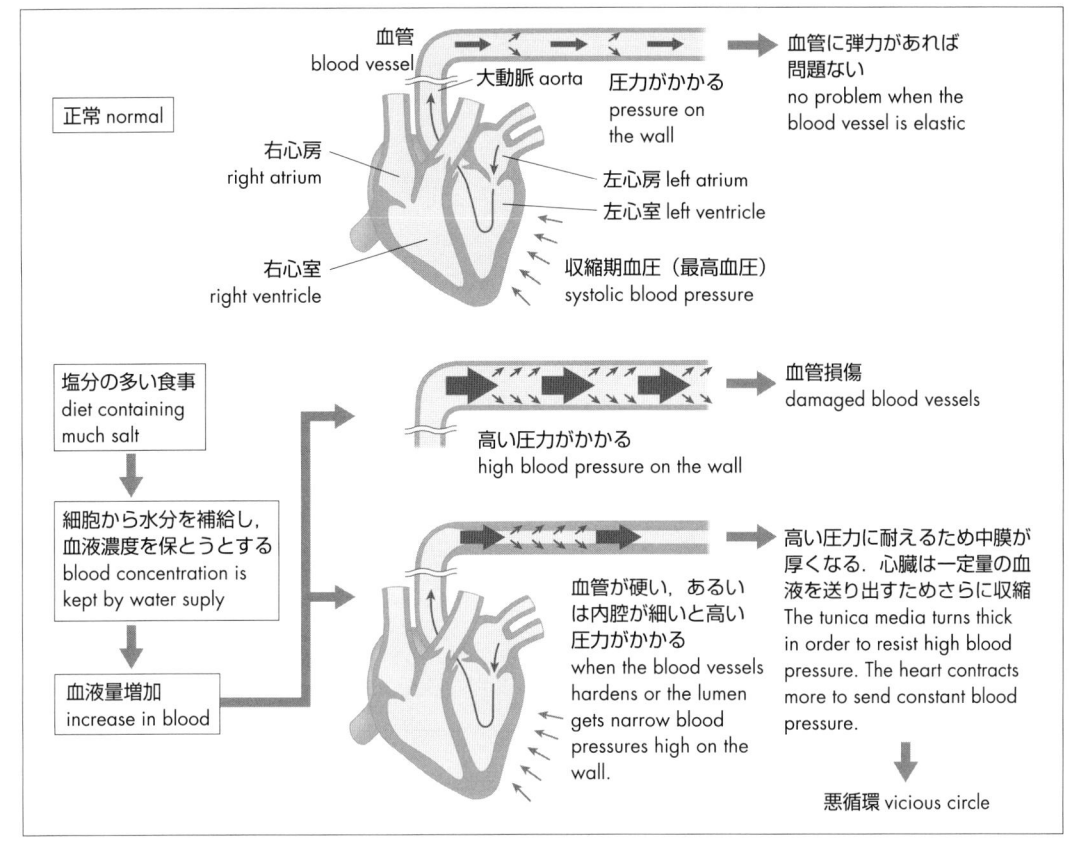

Figure 11 Mechanism of Hypertension（高血圧）

[ETIOLOGY]

Although essential hypertension is idiopathic, some persons are at a higher risk than others, including chronically stressed individuals, the obese, and those who favor a diet high in salt and saturated fats. Genetic factors have been assumed to play an important role in hypertension. Insulin resistance and hyperinsulinemia may be possible causes to hypertension.

Older persons, those with sedentary lifestyles, smokers, or those taking oral contraceptives also have a higher risk of hypertension.

[SIGNS and SYMPTOMS]

Persons with hypertension may remain asymptomatic for months or years or until vascular changes in the heart, brain, or kidneys occur. As they may suffer from other fatal cerebrovascular diseases or cardiac infarction, this pathological condition is sometimes called a "silent killer". The patient may exhibit vague symptoms, such as light-headedness, ringing in the ears (tinnitus), nocturia, a tendency to tire easily, and palpitations.

[DIAGNOSIS]

Blood pressure readings should be taken at least two times after the individual has rested. The definition of hypertension is agreed by the medical community (according to the Japanese Society of Hypertension) as any elevation of the systolic pressure (contraction) above 140 mmHg and of the diastolic pressure (relaxation) above 90 mmHg. It is important to realize that history of blood pressure readings must be kept for comparison, because blood pressure can vary according to various situations. Auscultation may reveal an abnormal heart sound (bruits). Electrocardiography (ECG) and chest x-ray films will help detect cardiovascular damage.

[TREATMENT]

Although there is no cure for essential hypertension, a change in lifestyle and diet, and the addition of antihypertensive drug therapy, can help control the condition. Diet management is also essential.

1) Medications
* Antihypertensive drugs
* Diuretics or vasodilators to relax and expand blood vessels

2) Dietary management
A nutritional diet low in salt and fat (low-sodium, low-fat diet) are essential as shown below. The patient should also avoid alcohol, caffeine, and nicotine, as well as refined carbohydrates and simple sugars. Nutritional and vitamin supplements may be helpful. If the patient is overweight should lose weight.

3) Nutritional standards
* Salt: 6 g/day
* Dietary fibers: 20-25 g/day
* Other nutrients: the diet based on the diet reference intakes
* Cholesterol in the case with heperlipidemia: less than 300 mg/day
* In cases with complications (e.g. obesity, dyslipidemia, diabetes mellitus): diet depends on therapy for each condition

REVIEW QUESTIONS

I Select the correct definition for each term.
1. palpitation 2. idiopathic 3. systolic pressure
4. blood pressure readings 5. Hg
   a) the number shown on sphygmomanometer used for measuring blood pressures
   b) Abbreviation of the chemical element mercury
   c) Relating to the any disease or condition for which cause is unknown
   d) Awareness that the heart is beating abnormally, due to stress or a disease
   e) The high point of blood pressure when the heart muscle contracts and pumps blood from the chamber into the arteries

II Write the appropriate term on the line.
1. It is divided into two types based on the causation: _____ hypertension and secondary hypertension.
2. Some hypertensive persons are at a higher risk than are others, including the obese, and those who favor a diet high in _____ and _____.
3. Persons with hypertension may remain _____ for months or years before symptomatic changes in the heart, brain, or kidneys occur.
4. Blood pressure readings should be taken at least _____ separate occasions after the individual has rested.
5. Diuretics or _____ relax and expand blood vessels.

III Write T for true, F for false on the line.
1. ____ Essential hypertension is persistent elevated blood pressure with apparent causes.
2. ____ Genetic factors have been assumed to play an important role in hypertension.
3. ____ The pathological condition of abnormal low blood pressure is sometimes called silent killer.
4. ____ The definition of hypertension is agreed by the medical community as any elevation of the diastolic pressure above 140 mmHg and of the systolic pressure above 90 mmHg.
5. ____ The patient with hypertension should also avoid alcohol, caffeine, and nicotine, as well as refined carbohydrates and simple sugars.

Nervous System Diseases and Disorders
神経系の疾患

Introduction to the Nervous System

What is the nervous system?

The human body's nervous system is an astonishing intricate neural network. This network of nerve cells is largely divided into two divisions: the central nervous system (CNS) and the peripheral nervous system (PNS). The CNS consists of the brain and spinal cord which consists of 8 pairs of cervical nerves, 12 pairs of thoracic nerves, 5 pairs of lumbar nerves, and 1 pair of coccygeal nerves. The

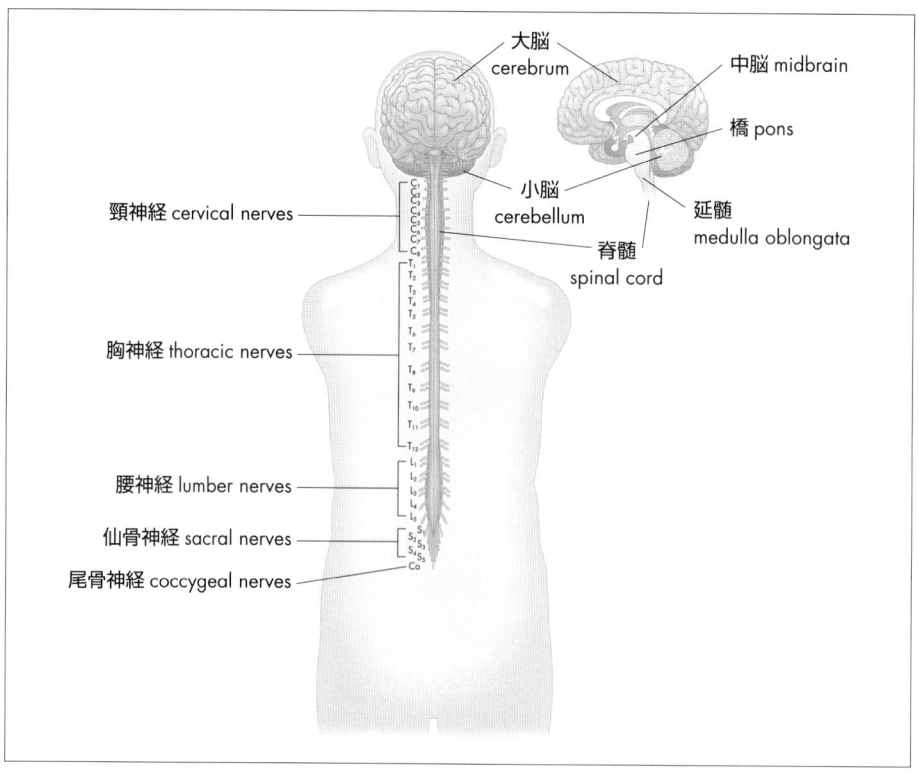

Figure 12　The brain stem and the spinal nerves（脳幹と脊髄神経）

brain has three major divisions: the cerebrum, the cerebellum, and the brain-stem. The PNS is composed of 12 pairs of cranial nerves from the brain, 31 pairs of spinal nerves from the spinal cord, all sensory nerves and the sympathetic and parasympathetic nerves. The sympathetic and parasympathetic nerves make up the third component, autonomic nervous system (ANS).

How does the nervous system work?

The entire nervous system functions to regulate and coordinate body activities and bring about responses by which the body adjusts to changes in its internal and external environment.

The CNS processes and stores sensory information and includes the parts of the brain governing consciousness. The CNS interacts with the second division of the nervous system, the peripheral nervous system. The autonomic nervous system (ANS) regulates involuntary muscle movements and the action of glands. The CNS together with PNS provide three general functions: sensory, integrative, and motor. The sensory function consists of receptors that monitor the body both externally and internally. The sensory receptors convert their information into nerve impulses, which are then transmitted via the PNS to the CNS and the signals are integrated. They are brought together, creating sensations and helping to produce thoughts and perceptions. The result is that we can make decisions and use motor functions to act on them.

1. Cerebrovascular Accident (Stroke)
脳血管障害（脳卒中）

　脳血管障害とは，脳に酸素とエネルギーを供給する脳動脈，さらにその分岐動脈が破れて出血，あるいは梗塞が生じた状態をいう．その結果，脳に重大な損傷が起き，またその影響によって軽度から重度の意識障害，身体麻痺，言語障害などが生じる．日本では，かつて死因の第1位であったが，最近では悪性新生物，心疾患に次いで第3位となり，2011年には肺炎が上まわり脳血管障害は4位となった．特に梗塞によるものが60％を占めている．卒中を可能な限り軽症に留めるには，特に初期の適切な対応が大切であるが，どのような状態の治療も適切な栄養療法の元に行われる．

KEY WORDS

Select the Japanese term most appropriate for each English term.
1. cardioembolic stroke　2. cerebral infarction　3. EEG　4. embolus
5. fatality rate　6. hemiparesis　7. ischemic stroke　8. MRI
9. occlusion　10. SPECT
a. 虚血性脳卒中　b. 心原性脳塞栓症　c. 磁気共鳴画像法　d. 死亡率
e. 脳梗塞　f. 脳波記録法　g. 塞栓
h. 単光子放射線型コンピュータ断層撮影　i. 不全片麻痺　j. 閉塞

[DESCRIPTION]

　A cerebrovascular accident or a stroke is a clinical syndrome marked by the sudden impairment of consciousness and subsequent paralysis. It is caused by occlusion or hemorrhaging of blood vessels supplying a portion of the brain. Deprived of adequate blood supply, the tissue in the affected portion of the brain becomes necrotic.

　There are two types of brain attack (1) ischemic stroke, in which a thrombosis or embolus interrupts the blood stream and (2) hemorrhagic stroke by the rupture of the blood vessel to the brain or subarachnoid membrane.

　In Japan, stroke used to be the major cause of death, but at the present, it is now the fourth most common cause of death after pneumonia. In addition, the higher fatality rate in cerebrovascular accident changed from hemorrhage stroke to cerebral infarction

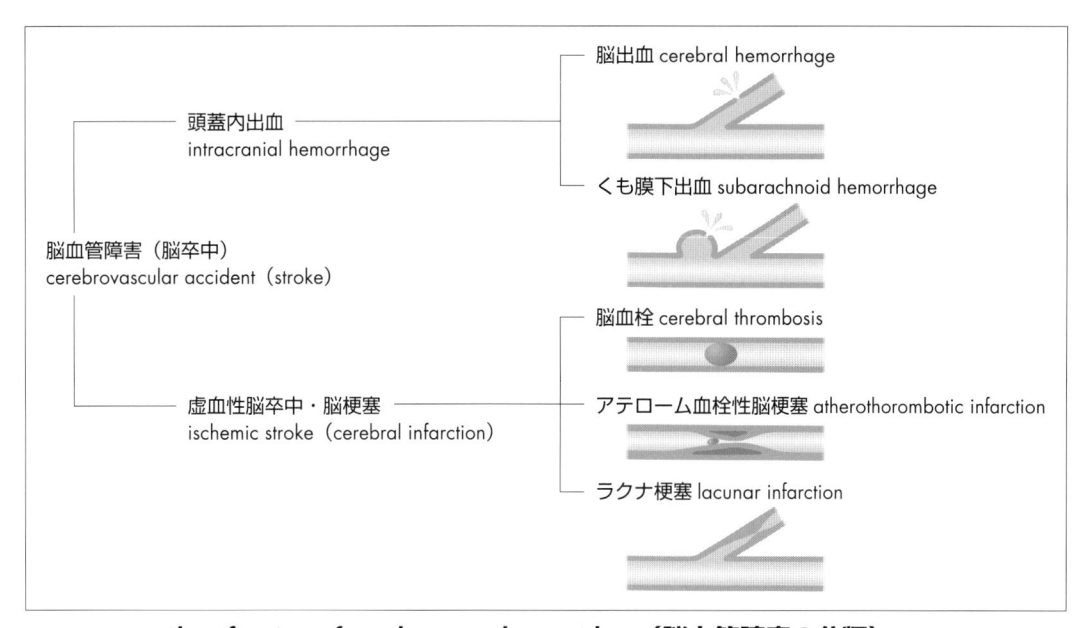

Figure 13 Classification of cerebrovascular accident（脳血管障害の分類）

(more than 60%).

[ETIOLOGY]

Causes of cerebrovascular accidents include life-style related illnesses such as diabetes mellitus, dyslipidemia and hypertension. Other risk factors include heart diseases, cerebral aneurysm, and a family history of atherosclerotic diseases, obesity, and a prior stroke. Habits, such as smoking, lack of exercise, a poor or high-fat diet, the use of oral contraceptives and even cocaine or other illegal drugs, also may be causes.

[SIGNS and SYMPTOMS]

The symptoms of strokes caused by an embolus or hemorrhage are often sudden in onset, whereas those caused by a thrombus may appear more gradually. Common symptoms include impaired consciousness ranging from stupor to coma, full and slow pulse, hemiparesis, and Cheyne-Stokes respiration characterized by a period of apnea lasting 10 to 60 seconds, followed by gradually increasing depth and frequency of respirations. Other symptoms

Cheyne-Stoks respiration：チェーンストークス呼吸：一回換気量が次第に増加，減少した後に呼吸停止．これを一周期（30秒〜2分）として反復する呼吸．うっ血性心不全，両側大脳半球から間脳の器質障害など，健常者でも高山の睡眠中にも見られる．John Cheyne（1777〜1836スコットランド），William Stoke（1804〜1878アイルランド）に由来．

include speech impairment (dysphasia), numbness, sensory disturbances, double vision (diplopia), poor coordination, confusion, and dizziness.

[DIAGNOSIS]

A comprehensive history-taking is a key to making a correct diagnosis: moreover, cerebral arteriography and electroencephlography (EEGs) are useful in confirming the diagnosis. Cranial computed tomography (CT) scans and magnetic resonnance imaging (MRI) often prove useful in pinpointing the affected portion of the brain and in helping to determine the mechanism that produced the stroke. Positron emission tomography (PET) and single-proton emission computed tomography (SPECT) are two other diagnostic tools used to study the blood flow and metabolic activity of brain lesions.

[TREATMENT]

Before an ambulance arrives, trying to talk to a person who seems to have lost consciousness is of primary importance to determine, if he/she is in a serious or mild condition. In the hospital, history taking should have priority over everything. The general treatment protocols include rest, drug therapy, and physical rehabilitation initiated as early as possible. Measures to prevent complications are important. All therapies for all types of a stroke should be given under the diet management.

1) Medications and other therapeutics

a) In the acute phase, treatment depends on the severity of the event and whether it was hemorrhagic or ischemic in origin as follows.

＊Anticoagulant: to improve cerebral circulation or to prevent and remove clots to control brain edema or cerebral infarction

＊Surgery, if necessary: for cerebral hemorrhage or subarachnoid hematoma

＊Physical rehabilitation: should be started for most stroke patients as early as possible to prevent physical and other disability

---

computed tomography (CT)：コンピュータ断層撮影法.　positron emission tomography (PET)：ポジトロン(陽電子放射)断層撮影法.

b) In the chronic phase, the following types of medicine will probably be prescribed.

*Antiplatelet agents (aspirin): for prevention of recurrent cerebral infarction

*warfarin potassium: for cardioembolic stroke to prevent thrombin in the heart

2) Dietary management

*energy requirement: 25–30 kcal/kg/day. The requirement varies according to changes in body weight. In infectious diseases, more should be supplied because of energy hypermetabolism.

*protein: 1.1 g/kg/day depending on age and kidney functions.
Aging persons should be supplied with sufficient protein because of their tendency to develop hypoproteinemia. However, in the case of renal hypofunction, the minimum is recommended.

*lipid: within 20–25% of total energy. Fatty acid intake should follow the dietary reference intakes.
In the case of hypercholesteremia, dietary cholesterol should be restricted to less than 300 mg/day.

Let's take a break.

再び，The You-Tell-'Em を．

You tell 'em, Cabbage,
　You've got the head.
言っておやりよ　キャベツさん
　頭じゃまけないよ，と．

このしゃれの落ちは cabbage です．古期フランス語の caboch（頭）から中期英語 cabache，そして現代の cabbage に変化したことによるものです．もうひとつの頭＝head の語源は，「鉢の形をした」という意味の古期英語です．そしてややこしいことに「キャベツ1個」は 'a head of cabbage' と言い，キャベツの芯は heart です．

さらに医学英語で頭は 'caput'（ラテン語）であり，encephalon＝brain は，cephalon（ギリシャ語の頭）の中（en-）にある脳です．さらにさらに，頭蓋骨は医学では cranium（ギリシャ語由来）があり，もうひとつの skull はスカンジナビア語からやってきて…えっ？ "I have a slight head ache." ですって？

REVIEW QUESTIONS

I Select the correct definition for each term.
1. CNS 2. paralysis 3. embolus 4. cerebrovascular accident
5. infarction

   a) The obstruction of the blood supply to the brain or an organ or the region of tissue, causing local death of the tissue
   b) Air clots, air bubbles, or small objects that have been carried in the blood flow and adhere to vessels causing blockage of an artery
   c) Loss of control in a muscle and function, such as sensation, secretion, or mental ability
   d) The sudden impairment of consciousness and subsequent paralysis caused by occlusion or hemorrhaging of blood vessels in the brain
   e) The part of the system of nerves that comprises the brain and spinal cord

II Write the appropriate term on the line.
1. There are two types of cerebral attack: _____ stroke, and _____ stroke.
2. Causes of _____ include life-style related illnesses such as diabetes mellitus, dyslipidemia and hypertension.
3. The symptoms of cerebrovascular accident are often sudden in _____, sometimes with sensory disorders, in contrast those caused by a _____ may appear more gradually.
4. Cranial CT =_____ scans and MRI often prove useful in pinpointing the affected portion of the brain.
5. All therapy for all types of stroke should be given under _____.

III Write T for true, F for false on the line.
1. ____ There is only one type of cerebrovascular accident which is very lethal.
2. ____ In Japan, the higher fatality rate of cerebrovascular accidents results from cerebral infarction.
3. ____ The symptoms of cerebrovascular accidents are often chronic, and have no relation sensory disorders.
4. ____ In the hospital, taking history should have priority over everything, to determine the treatment.
5. ____ Energy requirement for a cerebrovascular patient should be constant even if they gained weight.

2. Parkinson Disease　パーキンソン病

　パーキンソン病は，中脳黒質のドパミン分泌細胞に変調（ドパミン不足とアセチルコリンの増加）が生じ，著しい四肢の運動障害，摂食障害，認知障害などの機能低下を来たす神経変性の慢性疾患である．安静時振戦，筋固縮，無動，姿勢反射障害が身体症状の四徴といわれる．かつては発症後10数年で寝たきりとなったが，現在は薬物の飛躍的な効果によって社会生活の維持が可能になってきた．治療法の中心は薬物療法であるが，治療薬ドパミンの前駆物質の腸管吸収を助けるために，食事におけるたんぱく質量の制限を行う．そのほかの栄養素，栄養摂取量，咀嚼・嚥下障害の栄養管理も重要である．日本では好発年齢は50歳から65歳，有病率が人口10万人に100～150人，特定疾患に指定されている．

KEY WORDS

Select the Japanese term most appropriate for each English term.
1. absorption　2. bradykinesia　3. degeneration　4. motor dysfunction
5. neuropsychiatric disturbances　6. postural reflex disturbance
7. rigidity　8. substantia nigra　9. swallowing difficulties　10. tremor
a. 嚥下困難　b. 動作緩慢　c. 黒質　d. 固縮　e. 吸収　f. 振戦　g. 退化
h. 神経精神医学的障害　i. 姿勢保持反射障害　j. 運動機能障害

[DESCRIPTION]

　Parkinson disease is a chronic and degenerative disorder characterized by peculiar motor dysfunction. Most cases affect people from 50 to 60 years old. In the advanced stages, mental symptoms and signs such as apathy, anxiety, depression, mental and cognitive problems may arise. However, rapid progress in medicine makes patients able to maintain their social and daily lives longer than before. In Japan, the prevalence rate is around 100–150 per 100,000 population and the disease has been designated as an intractable disease since 1978.

[ETIOLOGY]

　The cause of degeneration in the nerve cells is unknown. Recent

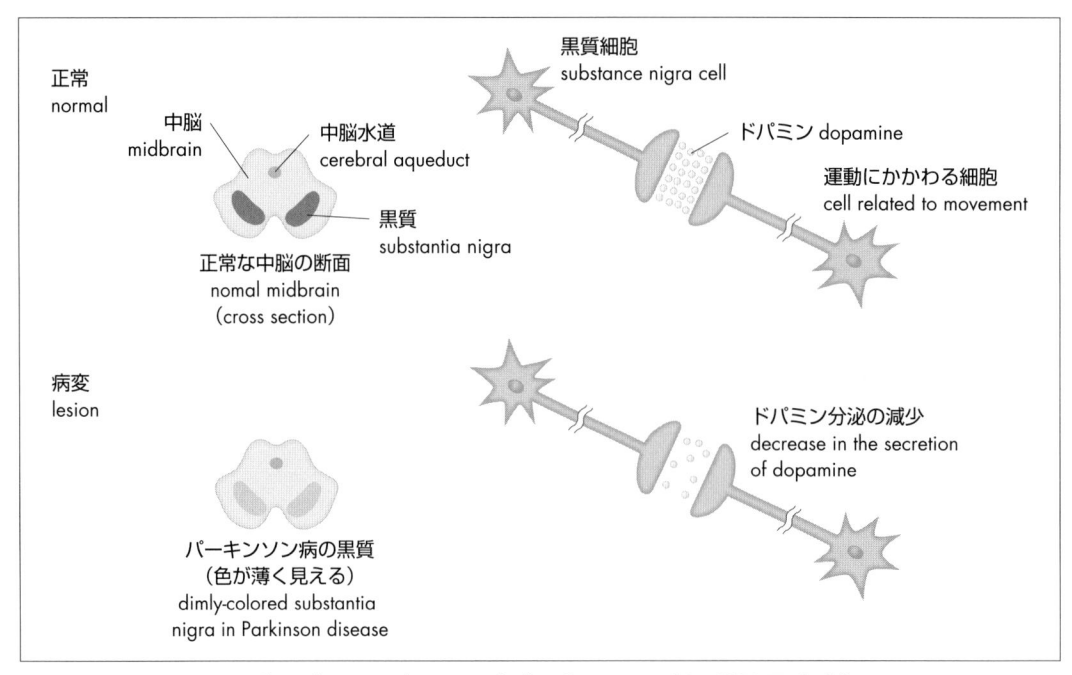

Figure 14 Lesions of Parkinson disease（パーキンソン病における病変）

studies show Lewy bodies, inclusion bodies within the dopamine cells, may be related to an insufficient formation and activity of dopamine in the substantia nigra (necessary neurotransmitter for brain cell functioning) in the region of the midbrain. They may produce the condition of specific motor dysfunction as well as neuropsychiatric disturbances.

Other suggested causes include genetics (juvenile), atherosclerosis, viral infections, head trauma, and chronic antipsychotic medication use.

[SIGNS and SYMPTOMS]

Symptoms typically may include "pill-rolling" tremors beginning in the fingers (resting tremor), abnormally muscular rigidity, slowness of movement (akinesia, bradykinesia) and balance difficulties (postural reflex disturbance). The patient's facial expression may appear fixed (masked face).

In the advanced stage, the patient also suffers from various neuropsychiatric disturbances; e.g. speech disorders, mental and

inclusion bodies：封入体.

cognitive and behavioral impairment, such as apathy, anxiety, and depression may arise.

[DIAGNOSIS]

Diagnosis is made on the basis of the medical history and a neurological examination. The characteristic symptoms mentioned above must be taken into consideration to distinguish Parkinson disease. If prescription of levodopa improves main motor symptoms except postural reflex disturbance, Parkinson disease is clinically diagnosed. The Unified Parkinson Disease Rating Scale (UPDRS) is useful for assessing both motor and non-motor symptom.

[TREATMENT]

The disease progression cannot completely be controlled; therefore, the goals are to alleviate the symptoms and to promote independence.

1) Medication

Medications such as L-dopa, dopamine agonists, MAO-inhibitors, COMT-inhibitors, amantadine, anticholinergic, droxidopa, zonisamide are prescribed (The 2011 guidelines for the treatment of Parkinson disease). If the drugs do not have any effect on the patient, surgery techniques may be tried to destroy part of the thalamus and limit involuntary movement.

2) Dietary management

Low-protein intakes over three meals should be given in order to help its easy absorption into the intestinal tubes, because the effectiveness of levodopa is reduced when taken together with protein. For a mild case, no special nutritional management is necessary, but a balanced diet based on the dietary reference intakes as well as periodic assessments are necessary to be attentive to. As Parkinson disease patients tend to retain food undigested in their stomach long, and also have swallowing difficulties, an appropriate diet should be prepared according to their condition.

The Unified Parkinson Disease Rating Scale：世界的なパーキンソン病統一スケール． MAO-inhibitors：monoamine oxidase inhibitor． COMT-inhibitors：cathechol-O-methyltransferase

REVIEW QUESTIONS

I Select the correct definition for each term.
  1. rigidity   2. tremor   3. degeneration   4. swallowing difficulties
  5. motor dysfunction
     a) A regressive change in the structure of cells or organs so that they no longer function satisfactorily
     b) Any loss or abnormality relating to muscular movement or activating nerves
     c) Condition of a person with stiff and nonflexible parts of the body
     d) The state of being hard to pass food or drink down
     e) An involuntary slight quivering movement in a part of the body

II Write the appropriate term on the line.
  1. Parkinson disease is a chronic and _____ disorder characterized by peculiar motor dysfunction.
  2. Symptoms of Parkinson disease typically may include _____, _____, bradykinesia and postural reflex disturbance.
  3. In the advanced stages, the Parkinson disease patient also suffers from various _____ disturbances.
  4. Lewy bodies, inclusion bodies within the dopamine cells, may be related to insufficient formation and activity of dopamine in the _____.
  5. _____ over three meals should be restricted in order to help its easy absorption into the intestinal tubes.

III Write T for true, F for false on the line.
  1.____ Parkinson disease is an acute and degenerative disorder with psychological disturbances which affect senior people.
  2.____ Lewy bodies within the dopamine cells may be related to an adequate formation and activity of dopamine in the substantia alba.
  3.____ The Parkinson disease patients suffer from various neuropsychiatric disturbances even in the early stage.
  4.____ Doctors identify Parkinson disease on the basis of the medical history and a neurological examination.
  5.____ High-protein intake over three meals should be restricted because levodopa works well when taken together with protein.

Unit 5 Respiratory System Diseases and Disorders
呼吸器系疾患

Introduction to the Respiratory System

What is the respiratory system?

The respiratory system consists of the nose, nasal cavities, pharynx (throat), larynx (voice box), trachea, and lungs. Lungs include bronchi, bronchioles and microscopic alveoli. The air passes through the nasopharynx (a part of the pharynx) into the larynx and the trachea, and food goes to the pharynx, then into the esophagus.

The trachea divides into the right and left main bronchi which enter the right and left lungs with pulmonary vessels together through an area called the hilum. Both bronchi divide further into smaller bronchi in each lung with numerous small bronchioles which eventually reach extremely tiny, thin walled air sacs called alveoli.

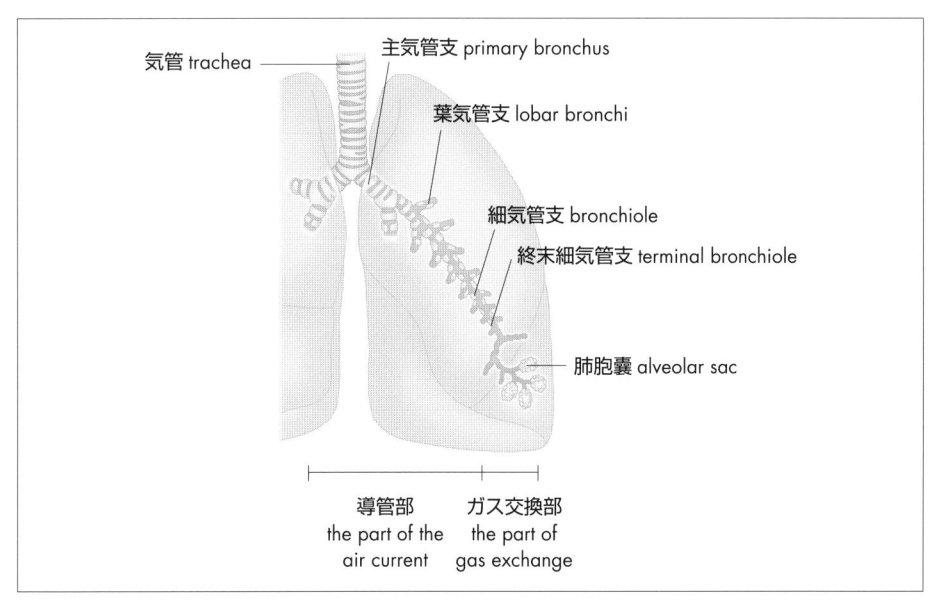

気管 trachea
主気管支 primary bronchus
葉気管支 lobar bronchi
細気管支 bronchiole
終末細気管支 terminal bronchiole
肺胞囊 alveolar sac
導管部 the part of the air current
ガス交換部 the part of gas exchange

Figure 15　The respiratory system （呼吸器系）

How does the respiratory system work?

The respiratory organs are the air passages from outside of the body to the terminal alveoli deep within lungs, where gas exchange takes place. Therefore, it may be said that alveolar function is the most important part of entire respiratory system.

A current of air containing oxygen comes mainly through the nostrils into the nasal cavity. Air moves ahead to smaller and smaller respiratory tracts and finally arrives at alveoli, small sacs like a cluster of grapes. As the number of alveoli is so huge (many times of the surface of the body if their total internal area were measured) and each is extremely thin walled, they enable large amounts of oxygen and carbon dioxide to be exchanged rapidly.

1. Chronic Obstructive Pulmonary Disease
慢性閉塞性肺疾患

　慢性閉塞性肺疾患は，生命維持に不可欠な酸素と二酸化炭素のガス交換が行われる肺胞に病変が起きる「肺気腫」と，気管支が侵される「慢性気管支炎」を含み，長期にわたる肺への損傷が原因で呼吸困難を来たす一連の症状を指す．緩やかに進行し，空気の流れが閉塞することで不可逆的息切れを生じ，慢性の咳，喀痰を伴う肺の炎症性疾患である．日本においては「タバコ病」と呼ばれるように，患者の約90％は喫煙者であり（受動喫煙も本疾患の起因となる），喫煙者の10～15％が発症するとされている．世界的にも日本においても死因の上位を占め，その予防と治療が大きな問題となっており，COPD国際ガイドライン（1997年）が作成され，改訂を重ねている．

KEY WORDS

Select the Japanese term most appropriate for each English term.
1. asthma　2. bronchiectasis　3. bronchitis　4. bronchodilator
5. dyspnea　6. pulmonary emphysema　7. pulmonary tuberculosis
8. respiratory quotient (RQ)　9. resting energy expenditure
10. spirometer
a. 安静時エネルギー消費量　b. 気管支炎　c. 気管支拡張症
d. 気管支拡張薬　e. 呼吸商　f. 呼吸困難　g. 肺活量計　h. 喘息
i. 肺結核　j. 肺気腫

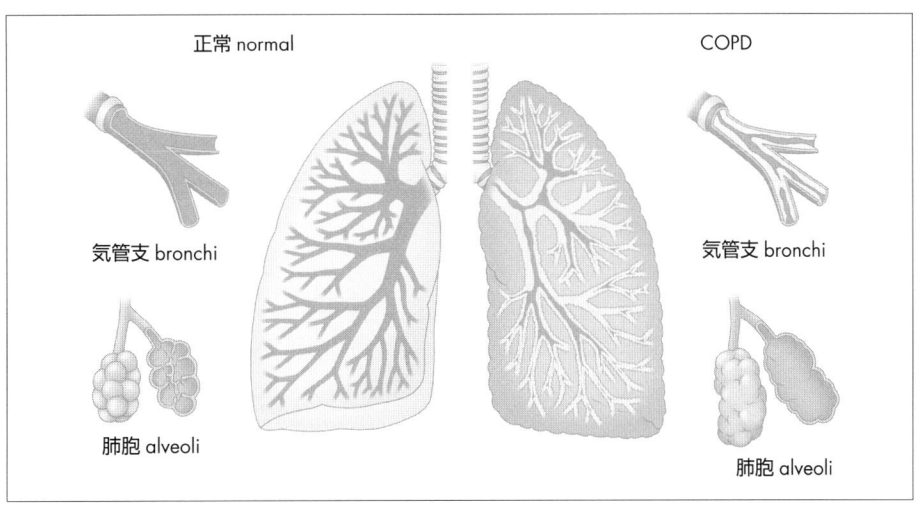

Figure 16　Chronic obstructive pulmonary disease（慢性閉塞性肺疾患）

[DESCRIPTION]

Chronic obstructive pulmonary disease (COPD) is a functional diagnosis given to any pathologic process that decreases the ability of the lungs and bronchi to perform their functions of ventilation. It is an umbrella term that includes chronic bronchitis and pulmonary emphysema. In COPD, air reaches the alveoli in the lungs during inhalation but may not be able to escape during exhalation.

Chronic bronchitis is inflammation of the bronchial mucosa. It is characterized by hypertrophy and hyperplasia of bronchial mucosal glands, damage to the bronchial cilia (hairlike extensions of cells), and narrowing of the bronchi.

Chronic pulmonary emphysema is permanent enlargement of the alveoli (the air spaces beyond the terminal bronchioles) resulting from destruction of alveolar walls. As a consequence of this destruction, the lungs slowly lose their normal elasticity causing difficulty in breathing.

[ETIOLOGY]

Diseases that may lead to COPD include emphysema, chronic bronchitis, chronic asthma, bronchiectasis, silicosis, and pulmonary tuberculosis. Smoking, prolonged exposure to polluted air, respiratory infections, and allergies are etiological factors in this disease. Occupational risk factors include exposure to textile dust fibers and certain petrochemicals. Evidence suggests that some forms of emphysema may be hereditary. In less common instances, emphysema is associated with a deficiency of α_1-antitrypsin which is a protein that plays a role in maintaining elasticity.

[SIGNS and SYMPTOMS]

COPD tends to develop insidiously, so no symptoms may be present initially. Later, a person may tire easily while exercising or doing strenuous work. Chronic cough, chest tightness, and increased sputum production may appear, followed by dyspnea on minimal exertion. As the disease progresses, the increase in airway resistance becomes greater. Weight loss, cyanosis, tachypnea, and wheezing may also be evident. Characteristic "barrel chest" is often seen in pulmonary emphysema.

[DIAGNOSIS]

A physical examination, a spirometer, chest x-ray films, pulmonary function tests, arterial blood gases, and electrocardiography are the procedures used to diagnose COPD, chronic pulmonary emphysema, and chronic bronchitis.

[TREATMENT]

Treatment is aimed at preventing further lung damage, relieving symptoms, and preventing complications. Persons diagnosed with COPD should be told not to smoke.

1) Medications

Bronchodilators may be used to open up the air passages in the lung, and antibiotics may be prescribed in the event of respiratory infections. Administration of oxygen may eventually be necessary.

2) Dietary management

In cases of malnutrition and progressive weight loss, proper nutritional guidance as well as nutrient supply treatment as follows is needed.

* Total energy intake: 1.5 times of the level at actual measured resting energy expenditure (REE) or 1.7 times that of estimated REE
* Prevention of amino acid imbalance: taking food rich in branched chain amino acids
* In a case of ventilatory failure: taking nutritional supplement which contains mainly lipid with low respiratory quotient (RQ)
* Making respiratory muscles contract: taking in enough phosphorus, potassium, calcium, magnesium
* Control over the sensation of abdominal distention or dyspnea: divided diet (4-6 times per day)
* In cases of pulmonary heart disease: taking low sodium diet

branched chain amino acid：分枝アミノ酸.　ventilatory failure：換気不全．気道，肺胞における吸気，呼気の換気が不十分な状態．

REVIEW QUESTIONS

I Select the correct definition for each term.
1. pulmonary emphysema   2. resting energy expenditure   3. bronchitis
4. spirometer   5. dyspnea
   a) Inflammation of the mucosa in the bronchi which typically causes bronchospasm and coughing
   b) Difficult breathing, usually associated with disease of the heart or lungs
   c) An instrument for measuring the air capacity of the lung
   d) A condition in which the alveoli of the lungs break down causing breathlessness and a lower oxygen level in the blood
   e) The amount of energy required for a 24-hour period by the strictly resting body

II Write the appropriate term on the line.
1. Chronic obstructive pulmonary disease (COPD) is an umbrella term that includes chronic _____ and pulmonary _____.
2. Chronic bronchitis is _____ of the bronchial mucosa.
3. _____, prolonged exposure to polluted air, respiratory infections, and allergies are predisposing factors in COPD.
4. To control the sensation of _____ or dyspnea, a patient should _____ their diet into 4-6 times per day.
5. The COPD patient with amino acid imbalance should take _____.

III Write T for true, F for fales on the line.
1.____ COPD is a comprehensive term that includes chronic bronchitis and pulmonary emphysema.
2.____ In COPD, air reaches the alveoli in the lungs during exhalation but may not be able to escape during inhalation.
3.____ Smoking is regarded as the only predisposing factor in COPD.
4.____ A patient with COPD should maintain 2 or 3 times of total energy intakes at actual measured resting energy expenditure (REE).
5.____ The COPD patient must take in only oxygen to make respiratory muscles contract.

Unit 6 Urinary System Diseases and Disorders
泌尿器系疾患

Introduction to the Urinary System

What is the urinary system?

The urinary system consists of a pair of kidneys, a pair of ureters, a bladder, and one urethra. The two kidneys are bean-shaped organs, situated on either side of the spine just above the line and against the muscles of the back. Each kidney is connected to the bladder by a long tube called a ureter. The bladder is a hollow, membranous sac,

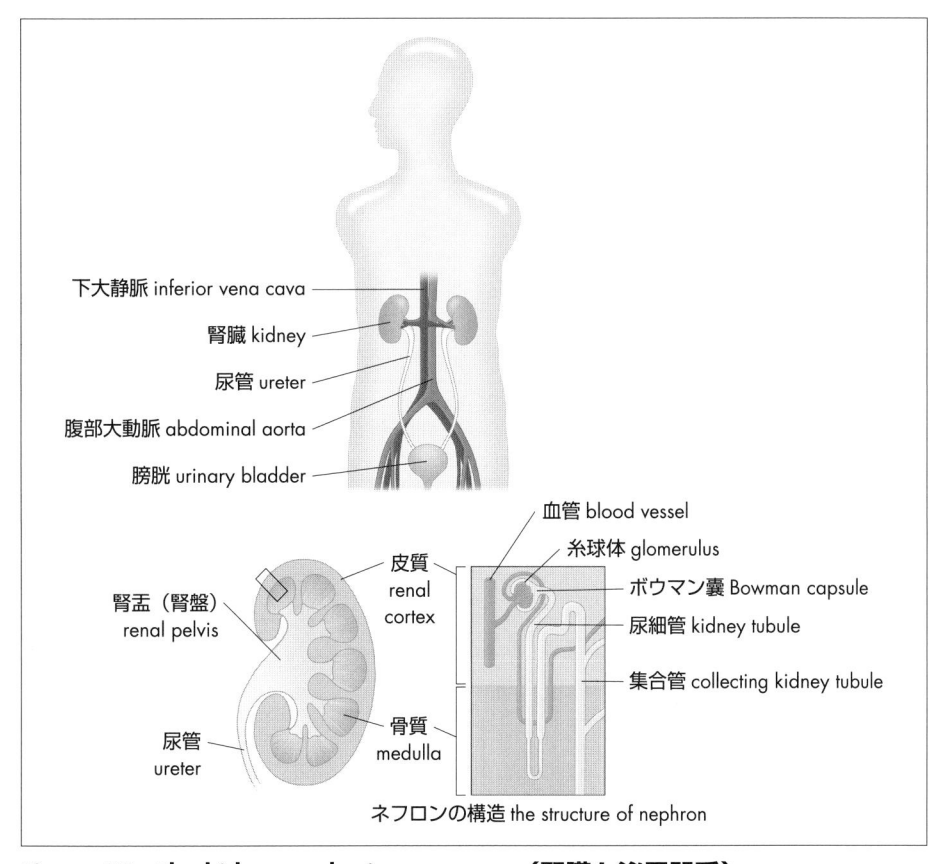

Figure 17 The kidney and urinary system (腎臓と泌尿器系)

situated centrally in the pelvis. And the urethra is the last urinary tube from the bladder to the outside of the body.

How does the urinary system work?

Thousands of metabolic processes in myriad body cells produce hundreds of waste products. The urinary system removes them by filtering and cleansing the blood as it passes through the kidneys. Another vital function is the regulation of the volume, acidity, salinity, concentration, and chemical composition of blood, lymph, and other body fluids. Under hormonal control, the kidneys continually monitor what they release into the urine to maintain a healthy chemical balance. Disorders of the system can be subtle, so urination-related symptoms should be promptly investigated.

Let's take a break.

今，breakの時間ですから，ADMEのE（excretion）へどうぞ．

ADMEとは，口腔から食道を無事通過した食塊が胃で撹拌され，一部が小腸からabsorbされ，栄養素となって血管へ，そして全身にdistributeされ，別の一部は肝臓の酵素によってmetabolizeされ，最後に尿管や直腸を通過してwastesとしてexcreteされるプロセスを，それらの頭文字から呼ぶ略語です．

医学にも，栄養学にも略語が数多くありますが，もとのスペリングを覚えるのも英語学習には効果的かも知れません．

さて，Eの場所の呼称にはいくつかあります．その昔，中学校時代に，我らが国語教師は生徒一人ひとりに聞きながら黒板に右から左へとEの場所を書いていったことを覚えています．我らの貧弱な語彙力はすぐに露呈して，感心しながらその多さに唖然としたものでした．その中にレストルーム，パウダールームはなかった．手水、ご不浄は大人たちが日常的に使っていましたが，雪隠，尿殿など不思議な言葉が印象的でした．ほかにも一穴，二穴…

英語にも標準的なtoilet, lavatory以外に，口語のloo（英），john（米）という隠語があり，そして，number one, number twoはおしっこ，うんちという幼児語です．どんな表現にしろ，適正な量と質の食物の摂取，器官と組織の活動，安定した心もちなどが，よき結果としてのbody wasteをもたらすことは言うまでもないでしょう．

1. End-stage Renal Diseases
(Chronic Renal Failure/Chronic Kidney Disease)
末期腎疾患（慢性腎不全）

腎不全とは，腎臓が血液中のクレアチニンや血中尿素窒素などの代謝性老廃物を排泄できなくなった状態をいう．同時に体液の量と配分や血液中の電解質の濃度を調節する能力も低下する．慢性的に腎不全になると，しばしば血圧が上昇，新しい赤血球の形成を促すホルモンを十分に産生できなくなり，赤血球数が減少し，貧血となり，成人も小児も骨が脆くなる．糸球体濾過量が減少し，ネフロンの約90％が失われ，乏尿・無尿となると，最終的には尿毒症を起こし腎透析療法・腎移植の対象になる．日本では最近，糖尿病腎不全が約50％を占め，次いで慢性糸球性腎炎が25％と増加している．通常，不可逆性であり，かつては治療が困難な疾患であったが，医療の進歩により腎機能の回復は可能となりつつある．

KEY WORDS

Select the Japanese term most appropriate for each English term.
1. azotemia   2. diabetic nephropathy   3. dialysis
4. glomerulonephritis   5. low-sodium diet   6. pyelonephritis
7. nephrosclerosis   8. oliguria   9. CKD   10. urinalysis
a. 乏尿症   b. 腎盂腎炎   c. 腎硬化症   d. 尿検査   e. 窒素血症
f. 糸球体腎炎   g. 低塩食   h. 糖尿病性腎症   i. 透析   j. 慢性腎不全

[DESCRIPTION]

End-stage renal disease (ESRD), sometimes referred to as chronic kidney disease (CKD) or chronic renal failure (CRF), is the gradual, progressive deterioration of kidney function. As the kidney tissue is progressively destroyed, the kidney loses its ability to excrete the nitrogenous end products of metabolism such as urea and creatinine, which accumulate in the blood, eventually reaching toxic levels. As kidney function diminishes, every organ in the body is affected, and dialysis or kidney transplantation is eventually needed for survival.

[ETIOLOGY]

In Japan, approximately 30-40% of chronic renal disease results from chronic glomerulonephritis. Recently, diabetic nephropathy is increasing as the main cause of this condition. Other causes include all kidney diseases (e.g. chronic pyelonephritis, nephrosclerosis, gouty kidney or glomerulonephritis, obstruction of the urinary tract and congenital anomalies such as polycystic kidneys) and vascular disorders, infections, medications, and toxic agents.

[SIGNS and SYMPTOMS]

The early signs are oliguria and the presence of nitrogenous compounds in increased amounts in the blood (azotemia); then electrolyte imbalance and metabolic acidosis follow. The patient may complain of progressive weakness and lethargy, weight loss, anorexia, diarrhea, hiccups, pruritus, and excessive formation and discharge of urine (polyuria). Patients with end-stage renal disease also may appear mentally confused and have pallid and scaly skin. The severity of signs and symptoms varies regarding the extent of the renal damage and residual function, any other underlying conditions, and the person's age.

[DIAGNOSIS]

The physical examination may detect one or more of the presenting signs and symptoms, along with hypertension. Blood testing typically reveals elevated serum creatinine, blood urea nitrogen, and potassium levels, along with decreased hemoglobin and hematocrit. Urinalysis may reveal proteinuria and urine that is highly diluted. The end-stage condition is determined by the following criteria of stages of CKD.

Stage G1	Slightly diminished function: kidney damage with normal or relatively high GFR (≥ 90 mL/min/1.73 m^2)
Stage G2	Mild reduction in GFR (60–89 mL/min/1.73 m^2) with kidney damage. Kidney damage is defined as pathological abnormalities or markers of damage
Stage G3a	Moderate reduction in GFR: 45–59 mL/min/1.73 m^2
Stage G3b	Moderate reduction in GFR: 30–44 mL/min/1.73 m^2
Stage 4	Severe reduction in GFR: 15–29 mL/min/1.73 m^2

Stage 5   Established kidney failure: GFR <15 mL/min/1.73 m^2
5D: Need for kidney dialysis
5T: Need for kidney transplantation

[TREATMENT]

Treatment is generally directed at relieving symptoms, retarding deterioration of remaining renal function, assisting the body compensating for the existing impairment, and guarding against complications. Dialysis or kidney transplantation may be attempted to prolong life. Furthermore, giving emotional support to the patient and family is of paramount importance.

1) Medication

Drugs below are prescribed depending on symptoms.
* Antiemetics to prevent or stop vomiting
* Angiotensin converting enzyme inhibitors (ACEIs), angiotensin II antagonists (ARBs) to control hypertension
* Erythropoietin and calcitriol, two hormones processed by the kidney (advanced stage)
* Phosphate binders (to control the serum phosphate levels)

2) Dietary management

Dietary restriction on nutrition includes;
* A high-calorie diet to avoid protein degradation by energy shortage (carbohydrate)
* A low-protein diet against uremic toxin (protein)
* A low-sodium diet not to worsen the condition of the glomeruli by hypertension (less than 7 g/day in the state of a high blood pressure measurements, 130/85 mmHg or higher)
* A low-potassium diet with vitamin supplements to prevent weakness in the muscle or neuropathy
* Water intake
  · no restriction in the state of only no oliguria, to prevent dehydration
  · urine volume on the previous day + 0.5 L to prevent pulmonary edema or heart failure caused by edema

130/85 mmHg：この数値は通常の血圧値よりも低い．

[DIALYSIS]

The blood of an individual experiencing acute or chronic renal failure typically contains high concentrations of metabolic waste products. Dialysis may be attempted to remove these wastes. In its broadest sense, dialysis is a process in which water-soluble substances are diffused across a semipermeable membrane. Most patients undergo 9 to 12 hours of dialysis per week, equally divided among several sessions. Factors determining the amount of dialysis include the patient's size, dietary intake, illnesses, and residual renal function. Three methods are currently used to dialyze the blood: peritoneal dialysis, hemodialysis, and continuous renal replacement therapy (CRRT).

continuous renal replacement therapy（CRRT）：持続的腎置換療法

REVIEW QUESTIONS

I Select the correct definition for each term.
1. oliguria   2. low-sodium diet   3. dialysis   4. kidney
5. glomerulonephritis

　a) A procedure for separating substances from a liquid, especially for removing soluble waste products from the blood of people with renal damaged

　b) Inflammatory changes in the glomeruli that are not caused by response to acute kidney infection

　c) Very small amounts of urine that may result in inefficient excretion of the products of metabolism

　d) A diet restricted to low amounts of sodium chloride, and other sodium salts, in the treatment of hypertension, heart failure.

　e) Each of a pair of organs in the abdominal cavity that remove waste products from the blood and produce urine

II Write the appropriate term on the line.
1. _____, sometimes referred to as chronic renal failure, is the gradual and progressive deterioration of kidney function.
2. In Japan, approximately 25% of chronic renal disease results from the state of chronic _____.
3. The patient may complain of _____ which means excessive formation and discharge of urine.
4. The _____ of an individual with renal failure usually contains high concentrations of metabolic waste products.
5. Dieticians will guide a _____ diet to the patient with uremic toxin.

III Write T for true, F for false on the line.
1. ____ Even if all organs of the body is affected by the kidney damages, dialysis is refrained for survival.
2. ____ In Japan, approximately 50% of chronic renal disease results from the state of acute glomerulonephritis.
3. ____ The severity of signs and symptoms varies depending on the extent of the renal damage and remaining function.
4. ____ Most clients undergo 9 to 12 hours of dialysis per month, equally divided among several sessions.
5. ____ The patient with end-stage renal failure needs to follow the diet therapy criteria which are divided into 5 grades.

2. Nephrotic Syndrome　ネフローゼ症候群

　ネフローゼ症候群は独立した疾患ではなく，通常，浮腫を伴い，低たんぱく血症，脂質異常，たんぱく尿の症状が診断基準となる病気である．しかし，浮腫は診断には必須ではない．この病気の主な原因は，糸球体腎炎からの移行であるが，他にも糖尿病性糸球体硬化症，全身性エリテマトーデス，アミロイドーシス，感染症などがある．食事療法の基本は，減塩，高エネルギー食，高たんぱく質食であるが，腎機能が低下し慢性腎不全の症状が見られると，低たんぱく質食となる．

KEY WORDS
Select the Japanese term most appropriate for each English term.
1. glomerulus   2. hemodialysis   3. high-protein diets
4. dyslipidemia   5. hypoalbuminemia   6. lipiduria   7. lupus
8. peritoneal dialysis   9. proteinuria   10. semipermeable membrane
a. 半透性膜   b. 高たんぱく食   c. 脂質異常症   d. 腹膜透析   e. 狼瘡
f. 糸球体   g. 血液透析   h. 脂質尿症   i. たんぱく尿
j. 低アルブミン血(症)

[DESCRIPTION]

　Nephrotic syndrome is a condition or a complex of signs and symptoms of the basement membrane of the glomerulus. The disease is characterized by severe proteinuria, often to the extent that the body cannot keep up with the protein loss (hypoalbuminemia). The disease is further characterized by excessive levels of fatlike substances called lipids in the blood (hyperlipemia), lipiduria and generalized edema.

[ETIOLOGY]

　Nephrotic syndrome may result from a variety of disease processes having the capacity to damage the basement membrane of the glomerulus. Between 70% to 75% of nephrotic syndrome cases result from some forms of glomerulonephritis. The syndrome also may arise as a consequence of diabetes mellitus, systemic lupus erythematosus, neoplasms, or reactions to drugs or toxins. The disease is occasionally idiopathic in origin.

[SIGNS and SYMPTOMS]

Edema is the most common symptom, and it may be either slow in onset or sudden. As body fluid accumulates, the patient may experience shortness of breath and anorexia. Abnormal accumulation of fluid in the peritoneal cavity (ascites), hypertension, pallor, and fatigue may result.

[DIAGNOSIS]

Nephrotic syndrome may be difficult to diagnose. Urinalysis may reveal proteinuria and increased waxy, fatty, granular casts. Blood serum tests may show decreased albumin level and increased cholesterol. Renal biopsy is important to establish a definitive diagnosis.

[TREATMENT]

1) Medication

Treatment is directed to symptoms, is supportive and aims to preserve renal function. The physician will attempt to manage the edema and hyperlipemia. Corticosteroids may be prescribed. Some

idiopathic：特発性(とくはつせい)＝固有の，原因不明の(agnogenic)　　granular cast：顆粒円柱

Table 4　Diet therapy criteria for patients with nephrotic syndrome (ネフローゼ症候群の栄養療法)

	total energy (kcal/kg*/day)	protein (kcal/kg*/day)	sodium (g/day)	potassium (g/day)	water
Except for minimal-change nephrotic syndrome	35	0.8	5	Increase or decrease depending on serum potassium level	No restriction**
Good therapeutic reactive minimal-change nephrotic syndrome	35	1.0–1.1	0–7	Increase or decrease depending on serum potassium level	No restriction**

*　standard body weight　**　restriction of water will be needed in case of severe refractory edema

patients will recover spontaneously.

2) Dietary management

High-protein diets, vitamin supplementation, and salt restriction may be prescribed. Any underlying disease or condition determined to be responsible for the nephritic syndrome must be treated as well.

According to the Japanese Society of Nephrology, the guidelines of the standard level of diet for clients of nephritic syndrome are as shown on the previous page.

Let's take a break.

今回はとんち問答を.
レストランで出されたスープに, fly が入っていたら？ もちろん, ウエイターを呼ぶはず. ところがそのウエイターからこんなふうに言われたら？

"Waiter, there's a fly in my soup."
"I've been looking for him all day."
「君, スープにハエが入ってますよ.」
「今日1日, 探していたのでございます.」

みなさんは, 謝らない彼に腹をたてるか, あるいは "A quick-witted waiter."（とんちの利くウエイター）と感心するか？ どちらでしょう. でも医学や生物学に実験体として貢献しているハエには申し訳ないのですが, 取り替えていただくより仕方がないでしょう.

ところで, その昔, 中学校の英語の授業で, fry と fly の発音に注意しなさい, と教えられたものでした. r と l では大違いです. どちらも日本人には発音が難しいのですが, 努々間違えないように.

REVIEW QUESTIONS

I Select the correct definition for each term.
1. proteinuria   2. urinalysis   3. hemodialysis   4. glomerulonephritis
5. glomerulus
   a) Acute inflammation of the kidney, typically caused by an immune response
   b) A process for separating substances and water from the blood by diffusion through a semipermeable membrane
   c) A cluster of capillaries around the end of a kidney tubule, where waste products are filttered
   d) The presence of abnormal quantities of protein in the urine, which indicate damage to the kidneys
   e) The identification and measurement of the chemical constituents of urine

II Write the appropriate term on the line.
1. The disease is characterized by severe _____, often to the extent that the body cannot keep up with the hypoalbuminemia.
2. Nephritic syndrome often results from some form of _____.
3. _____, vitamin supplementation, and salt restriction may be prescribed.
4. The patient with nephrotic syndrome undergoes most commonly _____.
5. A diagnosis of nephrotic syndrome is made after a series of tests, especially _____.

III Write T for true, F for false on the line.
1. ____ Nephritic syndrome is characterized by severe proteinuria, but not by hyperlipemia, lipiduria and generalized edema.
2. ____ Most cases of nephritic syndrome result from some forms of glomerulonephritis.
3. ____ Nephrotic syndrome shows a symptom of abnormal accumulation of fluid in the peritoneal cavity.
4. ____ Nephrotic syndrome may be easy to diagnose by the examination of blood serum test.
5. ____ In the case of minimal change of nephritic syndrome, a patient does not need limitation of salt.

Unit 7
Immune-related Diseases and Disorders
免疫系の疾患

Introduction to the Immune System

What is the immune response?

An ideal body would be free of disease. A careful study of body chemistry and cellular function reveals a blueprint for maintaining a disease-free state. The body is protected in three ways:

1. Normal body structures function to block the entry of germs through the use of tears, mucosa, intact skin, cilia, and body pH.
2. Inflammatory response rushes leukocytes to a site of infection, where invading organisms are engulfed in a process called phagocytosis.
3. A special immune response causes a protective reaction to a foreign antigen.

The body's immune system is both congenital and acquired. Congenital immunity is related to race, sex, and the individual's ability to respond.

The ability to generate an immune response is controlled by genetics. Immune response genes regulate B cell and T cell proliferation which influence resistance to infection and tumors. The immune response normally recognizes its own body cells, thereby preventing self-damage to tissue.

Although this complex system to protect the body is an example of the disease-free design of the body, the immune response can malfunction. Immunologic malfunctions are classified as (1) allergy, when the immune response is inappropriate; (2) autoimmunity, when the immune response is misdirected; and (3) immunodeficiency, when the immune response is inadequate.

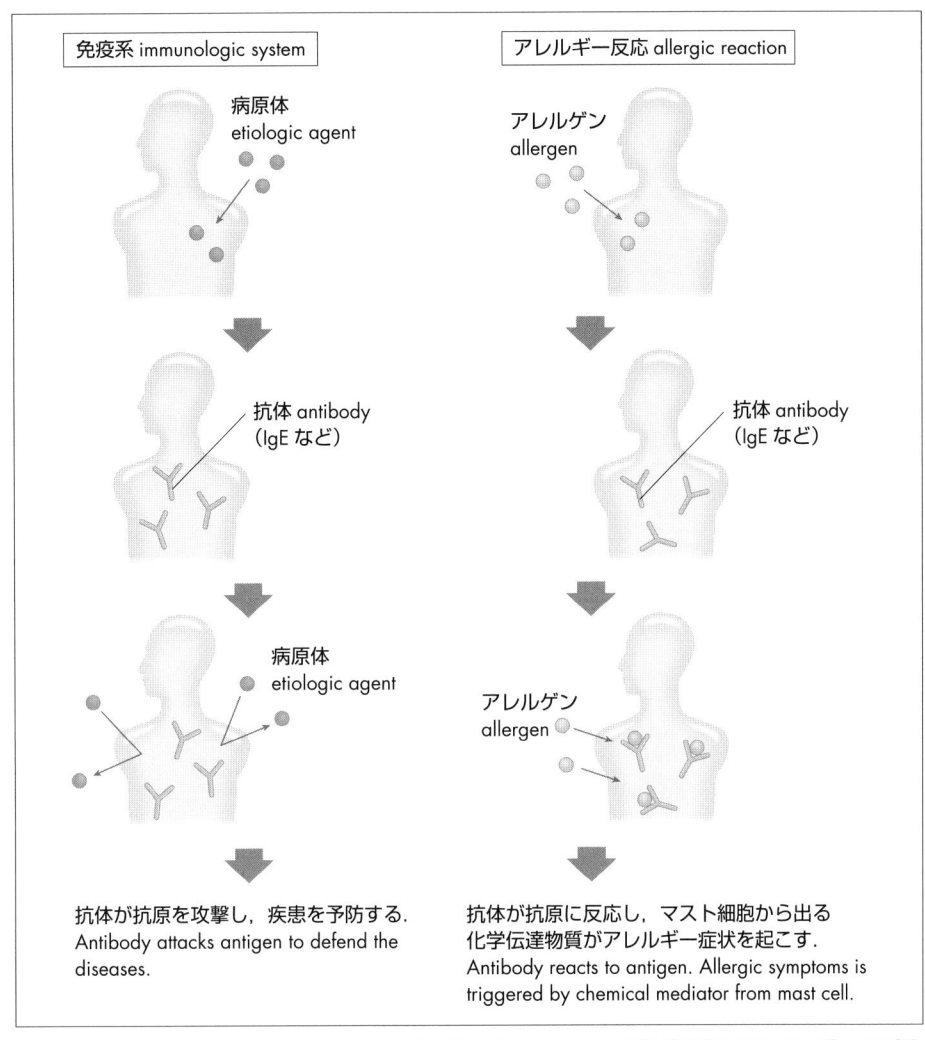

免疫系 immunologic system	アレルギー反応 allergic reaction
病原体 etiologic agent	アレルゲン allergen
↓	↓
抗体 antibody（IgE など）	抗体 antibody（IgE など）
↓	↓
病原体 etiologic agent	アレルゲン allergen
↓	↓
抗体が抗原を攻撃し，疾患を予防する． Antibody attacks antigen to defend the diseases.	抗体が抗原に反応し，マスト細胞から出る化学伝達物質がアレルギー症状を起こす． Antibody reacts to antigen. Allergic symptoms is triggered by chemical mediator from mast cell.

Figure 18　The immune system and allergic response（免疫系とアレルギー反応）

1. Food Allergy　食物アレルギー

　食物アレルギーは，特定の食物に含まれるたんぱく質によって免疫反応を起こす疾患をいう．さまざまな症状が現れるが，即時型（食後，すぐ反応が現れる）にはじんましん，痒み，発疹などの皮膚症状や，呼吸器の喘鳴，せきなどがみられる．遅延型（食後48時間経過後）では免疫細胞がたんぱく質を抗原として記憶し，再び同じたんぱく質が体内に入ると免疫反応が起き炎症を起こす．基本的治療は原因の食物を摂取しないことである．そのため，アレルゲンを特定するためのいくつかの方法が取られるが，長期にわたるテストや予想されるアレルゲンを排除する除去食などに患者は苦痛を伴うので，周囲の理解と協力が必要とされる．生命にかかわる全身症状のアナフィラキシーに対しては，アドレナリン筋肉注射が緊急に必要とされる．食物アレルギーの三大原因は，卵，牛乳，小麦であるが，日本においては消費者が食品摂取の際に前もって危険を知るために，厚生労働省は25の特定原材料を，そのうち7品目の表示を義務づけ，18品目の表示を奨励している．

KEY WORDS

Select the Japanese term most appropriate for each English term.
1. anaphylaxis　2. antiallergic drug　3. antibody　4. antigen
5. elimination diet　6. immunoglobulin E　7. mandatory labeling
8. oral challenge test　9. specified ingredients　10. hives
a. 経口負荷試験　b. 抗アレルギー薬　c. 表示指定　d. 抗原　e. 除去食
f. 免役グロブリンE　g. アナフィラキシー　h. 特定原材料　i. 抗体
j. じんましん

[DESCRIPTION]

　Food allergy refers to immunological reactions against food antigen that sometimes cause serious illness and death. This response is mediated by immunoglobulin E (IgE) to protect the body against abnormal or foreign body called antigens. Once an antigen enters the body, persons with allergic diathesis respond to the antigen which causes various allergic symptoms in the body. However, it is necessary to distinguish these and other non-allergic responses which include causes by food poisoning by toxins and food intolerability due to defects in digestive enzymes because the latter two do not involve the immune response.

In Japan, 27 'Specified ingredients' are designated by the Ministry of Health, Labor and Welfare to label on foods ; 7 items as "mandatory labeling" (specified ingredients) and 20 as "items corresponding to specified allergy-related ingredients".

[ETIOLOGY]

Food allergies are commonly triggered by proteins in food. Many different foods are responsible for allergic reactions. As mentioned above, 7 items (shrimp/prawns, crab, wheat, buckwheat, eggs, milk and peanuts), and 18 other specified items (abalone, squid, salmon roe, oranges, kiwi fruit, beef, walnuts, salmon, mackerel, soybeans, chicken, bananas, pork, "matsutake" mushrooms, peaches, yams, apples, gelatin, sesame and cashew nuts) are regarded as common dietary allergens.

In children, eggs and milk are common food allergens. Food allergies may affect children under age 5, but about 10% of them lose their allergic reactions without any special treatment as they grow up.

In addition, individual allergic disposition is considered as a factor that triggers food allergies in both children and adults.

[SIGNS and SYMPTOMS]

In immediate hypersensitivity, a food allergy occurs soon or within several hours after eating particular foods. The reaction and severity depends on the individual, age and ingredient in food. Symptoms like itching, rashes and edema appear on the skin. General symptoms such as diarrhea and abdominal pains in the digestive ducts, asthma or dyspnea in the respiratory organs commonly occur. In the case of anaphylaxis, low blood pressure, difficulty in breathing, or consciousness disturbance may be life-threatening.

In an infant, the first symptom of a food allergy may be atopic dermatitis. Then nausea, vomiting and diarrhea may follow. Such

---

food poisoning：食中毒. 25 'Specified ingredients'：加工食品に含まれるアレルギー物質の表示として，特定原材料（表示義務）7品目，特定原材料に準ずる（表示の推奨）18品目が，食品衛生法により定められている． immediate hypersensitivity：即時型アレルギー. atopic dermatitis：アトピー性皮膚炎．

symptoms may subside gradually.

[DIAGNOSIS]

First of all, doctors will start taking the patient's history to find a food allergen. Then, some of the following might be performed.

a) Skin tests: a small amount from an extract of the suspected food allergen is put on the skin of the arm or back. However, this test alone may not satisfy to confirm a food allergen.

b) Oral challenge test: the individual is given small but increasing amounts of the suspected allergens and is observed while eating them. If no symptoms appears, there is not a food allergy.

c) Elimination diet: suspected foods are removed from the patient's diet for a week or two and reinstated if there are no allergic symptom (See the next).

[TREATMENT]

1) Medication

Antihistamines can be helpful to reduce a minor allergic reactions (e.g. itching, hives or swelling), but not for treatment for severe food allergies.

In case of shock, epinephrine or steroids are necessary for immediate treatment. An epinephrine auto-injector is often carried by individuals with severe food allergies to counteract anaphylactic emergencies.

Sodium cromoglicate may also be used as an antiallergic drug.

2) Dietary management

As a general rule, there are two types of elimination diet; complete and incomplete. As elimination therapy is very stressful for the patient, especially school children, consideration of the nutritional and mental situation of the patient is needed in cooperation with his/her family as well as teachers concerned. Arrangements that require attention are as follows.

3) Points requiring attention

a) In a case of a complete elimination diet, pay attention to processed

---

hives：じんま疹＝urticaria, nettle rash.　swelling：腫脹.　epinephrine：エピネフリン製剤＝adrenaline アドレナリン製剤.　sodium cromoglicate：クロモグリク酸ナトリウム.

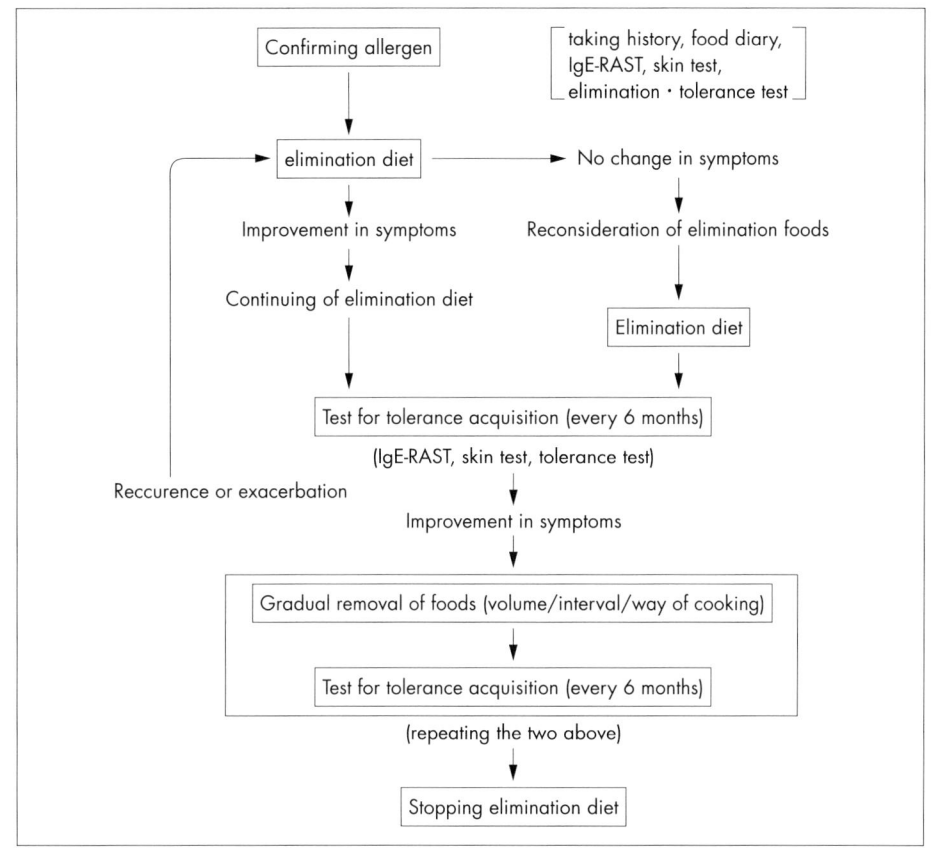

```
                    ┌─────────────────────┐   ┌taking history, food diary,┐
                    │ Confirming allergen │   │IgE-RAST, skin test,        │
                    └─────────────────────┘   └elimination・tolerance test┘
                              ↓
                    ┌──────────────────┐
              ┌────→│ elimination diet │─────→ No change in symptoms
              │     └──────────────────┘                ↓
              │               ↓                Reconsideration of elimination foods
              │     Improvement in symptoms              ↓
              │               ↓                ┌──────────────────┐
              │     Continuing of elimination diet  │ Elimination diet │
              │               ↓                └──────────────────┘
              │     ┌──────────────────────────────────────┐
              │     │ Test for tolerance acquisition (every 6 months) │
              │     └──────────────────────────────────────┘
              │          (IgE-RAST, skin test, tolerance test)
     Reccurence or exacerbation        ↓
                         Improvement in symptoms
                                  ↓
              ┌──────────────────────────────────────────────────┐
              │ Gradual removal of foods (volume/interval/way of cooking) │
              └──────────────────────────────────────────────────┘
                                  ↓
              ┌──────────────────────────────────────────┐
              │ Test for tolerance acquisition (every 6 months) │
              └──────────────────────────────────────────┘
                         (repeating the two above)
                                  ↓
                    ┌─────────────────────────┐
                    │ Stopping elimination diet│
                    └─────────────────────────┘
```

Figure 19　Arrangements of elimination diet（除去食療法実施の手順）

foods (e.g. 27 specified ingredients designated by the Ministry of Health, Labor and Welfare/food additives), and also to usage of cookware.

b) Denaturing the allergic food by heat treatment to prevent its allergic reaction in the body.

c) Refrain from excessive intake of the same food including chemical substances such as histamine (e.g. spinach, eggplant) or serotonin (e.g. banana, pineapple).

d) Foods of the same family which produces cross-reaction (e.g. orange or lemon) in the diet need to be confirmed.

e) Mothers need to restrict their food with breastfeeding.

f) Introduce alternative meal with consideration for the patient's balanced nutrition and taste.

g) Refrain from drinking excessive alcohol.

h) Consider the patient's stress caused by elimination diets and

restriction on his/her participation in the social activities.
i) Reinforce the diet therapy together with oral disodium cromoglicate (DSCG) to inhibit absorption of allergen.

Let's take a break.

　再びサラダに戻ります．明治の文豪，夏目漱石の『草枕』では，「西洋の食べ物は色がよくない，サラドと赤大根だけはいい」と登場人物のひとりがサラドと英語読みで言っています．しかし，サラダもサラドも昔のラテン語sal（塩）が語源です．おそらく当時のローマ人たちは生野菜に塩を振りかけて食したのでしょう．フランス語salade，イタリア語insalata，ドイツ語Salat，ポルトガル語saladaもすべてsalからサラダになりました．日本語のサラダはポルトガル語の読み方からでしょう．

　そういえば，a green saladは「青野菜サラダ」です．前のbreakで触れたcirrhosisがそうであるように医学英語には色彩用語がよく含まれています．思いつくまま例を挙げておきましょう．

jaundice：黄疸［フランス語jaune＝黄色］
xanthoma diabeticorum：糖尿病性黄色腫［ギリシャ語xanthos＝黄色］
melanoma：黒色腫［ギリシャ語melas＝黒色］
substantia nigra：黒質［ラテン語niger＝黒色］
poliomyelitis：ポリオ［ギリシャ語polios＝灰色］
leukemia：白血病［ギリシャ語leukos＝白色］
albumin：アルブミン［ラテン語albus＝白色］
chlorophil：葉緑素［ギリシャ語khloros＝緑色］

　色は色々です．

REVIEW QUESTIONS

I Select the correct definition for each term.

1. elimination diet   2. hives   3. anaphylaxis   4. specified ingredients
5. antigen

   a) An extreme, often life-threatening allergic reaction to some foods or something
   b) A foreign substance that induces a sensitive immune responsiveness in the body, especially the production of antibodies
   c) A diet designed to detect food that is causing an allergic reaction in the body.
   d) Foods designated by the Ministry of Health, Labor and Welfare as materials containing allergens
   e) A rash of round, red wells of the skin that itch intensely, sometimes with dangerous swelling.

II Write the appropriate term on the line.

1. Food allergy refers to _____ against food antigen that sometimes causes serious illness and death.
2. In Japan, _____ designates to label on 7 items of foods as "mandatory labeling" and 20 as "items corresponding to specified ingredients."
3. Food allergies can trigger a life-threatening _____ which occurs in a hypersensitive individual.
4. _____ is a way to confirm an allergen by removing a suspected food from the patient's diet for a week and replacing it again.
5. As a general rule, there are two types of elimination diet; _____ and _____.

III Write T for true, F for false on the line.

1. ____ Food allergy refers to a chemical response to food that sometimes causes a serious change in the living body.
2. ____ Food allergies are commonly triggered by proteins in many different foods.
3. ____ In Japan, the Ministry of Health, Labor and Welfare designates 20 items of food for labeling as mandatory labeling.
4. ____ In the case of anaphylaxis, low blood pressure and difficulty in breathing, are not life-threatening.
5. ____ A general treatment of food allergy is to remove a food suspected as allergen.

Unit 8 Metabolic Diseases and Disorders
代謝疾患

Introduction to Metabolism

What is metabolism?

Metabolism consists of the chemical and physical processes (absorption, synthesis and decomposition of chemical substances) crucial to life of all living organisms, not just humans. After food is eaten, it is absorbed, especially in the small intestine; proteins are converted into amino acids, fats into fatty acids, and carbohydrates into simple sugars (for example glucose) by chemical digestive agents called enzymes. Blood carries these compounds with other enzymes to the cells in which two phases of metabolism, anabolism and catabolism, take place at the same time.

During anabolism, small molecules are changed into larger and more complex molecules of carbohydrate, protein and fat. Structural proteins act to repair and replace the tissue of the body. Functional proteins contain enzymes which speed up chemical reactions; antibodies which either destroy the abnormal or foreign material or make it harmless; and most hormones, which regulate various

anabolism：constructive metabolism. 同化.

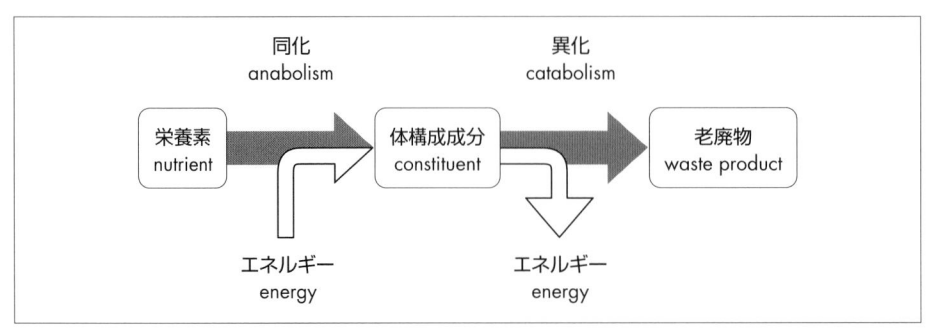

Figure 20 Mechanism of metabolism （代謝のメカニズム）

processes. Cells also change fatty acids and glucose to stored energy, each in the form of adipose tissues and glycogen respectively, for later use.

During catabolism, large molecules (mostly carbohydrate and fats) are broken down in cells and released, and provide energy and heat to the body as fuels. Catabolism also functions in the process of removing the waste products from the body through the skin, kidneys, and intestines.

Metabolic disorders

A sequence of chemical reactions takes place through metabolic pathways, mostly enzyme-dependent. Most metabolic disorders occur somewhere along these pathways, involving either abnormal levels of enzymes or hormones which regulate these pathways, or problems with the functioning of those enzymes or hormones. They can be congenital because of a defect in a single gene or acquired resulting from endocrine organ disease or liver failure.

As they are usually asymptomatic, most metabolic disorders in themselves are not harmful to life. However, if the abnormal condition prolonged, for example, excess glucose in blood causes diabetes, and diabetes leads to serious problems such as blindness, peripheral vascular diseases or kidney diseases. In hyperlipidemia, a gradual increase in cholesterol in blood accelerates arteriosclerosis, which sometimes results in cardiac infarction or cerebral thrombosis.

Thyroxin, a hormone secreted from the thyroid gland, controls the rate of metabolism, and hormones secreted in the pancreas determine the metabolic pathway. Dietitians determine a person's energy by measuring the basal metabolic rate (BMR), which is the rate of metabolism at rest, because the BMR differs according to build, age and sex.

catabolism：destructive metabolism. 異化.

1. Dyslipidemia　脂質異常症

　脂質異常症は，血液中に脂質(特にコレステロールと中性脂肪)が過度に蓄積する，あるいは不足する状態をいう．特に，前者は動脈硬化を，ひいては日本人の死因の上位を占める心疾患や脳卒中などを引き起こすリスクが高いために，その対策が国民的課題となっている．日本では診断基準が変更され(動脈硬化学会2007年)，従来の高脂血症と低リポたんぱく血症を包含し，脂質異常症と呼ばれるようになった．必ずしも症状を伴わないが，コレステロール値の検査によって異常が診断される．治療は，食事療法が主であり，薬物療法，運動療法とあわせて行われる．

KEY WORDS

Select the Japanese term most appropriate for each English term.
1. atherosclerosis　2. cerebrovascular disease
3. coronary artery disease　4. genetic makeup
5. high density lipoprotein cholesterol　6. hypercholesterolemia
7. hypertriglyceridemia　8. lipid-lowering drug
9. low density lipoprotein cholesterol　10. unsaturated fatty acid
a. 不飽和脂肪酸　b. 遺伝体質(遺伝子構造)　c. 粥状硬化　d. 冠動脈疾患
e. 高比重(高密度)リポたんぱくコレステロール　f. 高コレステロール血症
g. 高トリグリセリド血症　h. 脳血管障害　i. 脂質降下薬
j. 低比重(低密度)リポたんぱくコレステロール

[DESCRIPTION]

　Dyslipidemia is grouped into two categories: hyperlipidemia and hypolipoproteinemia. In developed countries, most dyslipidemia are hyperlipidemias; an abnormal excess of any or all fatty substances (e.g. cholesterol, or triglycerides) in the blood which attaches to proteins (fat-protein complexes) and travel in the blood circulation. Both low density lipoprotein (LDL) and high density lipoprotein (HDL), the fat-complex lipoproteins, are involved in hyperlipidemia.

　In Japan, the diagnostic criteria of dyslipidimia has been changed since 2007 by the Japan Atherosclerosis Society. (see DIAGNOSIS)

[ETIOLOGY]

Factors that increase the risk of hyperlipidemia (hyperlipoproteinemia) include having close relatives who have had hyperlipoproteinemia, being overweight, consuming a diet high in saturated fats and cholesterol, being physically inactive, and consuming a moderate to excessive amount of alcohol. A person's genetic makeup, some disorders (diabetes, kidney failure, obstructive liver disease, hypothyroidism), and uses of drugs (estrogen, oral contraceptives, corticosteroids, thiazide diuretics) can also cause hyperlipidemias.

[SIGNS and SYMPTOMS]

High lipid levels in the blood usually cause no symptom. The risk of developing atherosclerosis increases as cholesterol levels increase. Atherosclerosis can affect the arteries that supply blood to the heart (causing coronary artery disease), those that supply blood to the brain (causing cerebrovascular disease), and those that supply blood to the rest of the body (causing peripheral disease). However, having a very low cholesterol level may not be healthy either. In parts of the world such as China and Japan where the average cholesterol level is 150 mg/dL, coronary artery disease is less common than it is in countries such as the United States.

[DIAGNOSIS]

The total cholesterol level is a general guide to the risk of atherosclerosis with assessment of diabetes, hypertension and obesity. Levels of LDL cholesterol, HDL cholesterol, and triacylglycerol are measured in blood after fasting at least 12 hours

Table 5 Diagnostic criteria of dyslipidemia (脂質異常症診断基準)

1) hypercholesterolemia low density lipoprotein cholesterol (LDL-C)	≥ 140 mg/dL
2) hypolipoproteinemia high density lipoprotein cholesterol (HDL-C)	< 40 mg/dL
3) hypertriglyceridemia triacylglycerol	≥ 150 mg/dL

(Japan Atherosclerosis Society: Prevention of atherosclerotic cardiovascular diseases 2007)

Table 6 The basic diet standard for a patient with dyslipidemia（食事療法の基本）

1st step: Making proper intakes of total energy, balanced nutrients and cholesterol
1) proper total energy intake 　　proper energy intake = standard body weight × 25–30 (kcal) 　　＊standard body weight = [height (m)] × [height (m)] × 22 2) balanced intakes of nutrients 　　carbohydrate: 60% 　　protein: 15–20% (more fish meat and soybean than animal meat or chicken) 　　fat: 20–25% (less animal meat fat and chicken fat, more vegetable fat and fish fat) 　　cholesterol: less than 300 mg/day 　　dietary fiber: more than 25 g 　　alcohol: less than 25 g 　　others: vitamins (C, E, B_6, B_{12}, folic acid etc.) and vegetables and fruits containing much polyphenol)　(a desirable intake in fruits: within 80–100 kcal/day because of containing much monosaccharide)
[When the serum lipid does not reach the target levels, the patient will progress next]
2nd step: Limiting diet therapy according to the types of cholesterolemia
1) hypercholesterolemia 　　tightening control on fat intake: less than 20% fat energy intake in total energy intake 　　limiting cholesterol intake: less than 200 mg/day 　　proper intakes of saturated and unsaturated fatty acid: at a rate of saturated fatty acid: monoenoic unsaturated fatty acid: polyunsaturated fatty acid = 3 : 4 : 3 2) hypertriglyceridemia 　　stopping drinking alcohol 　　limiting carbohydrate intake: less than 50% carbohydrate energy intake in total energy intake 　　limiting monosaccharide intake as much as possible: if possible only with an intake of 80–100 kcal from fruits 3) hypercholesterolemia with hypertriglyceridemia 　　practice of 1) and 2) above 4) hyperchylomicronemia 　　limiting fat intake: less than 15%

(Japan Atherosclerosis Society: Prevention of atherosclerotic cardiovascular diseases 2007)

before the blood sample is taken. In Japan, dyslipidemia has been diagnosed by the volume of cholesterol on the previous page according to the new diagnostic criteria since 2007.

[TREATMENT]

　Usually, the best treatment for people who have dyslipidemia is to change their life style, that is, to maintain an appropriate food habit, stop smoking, and increase physical activity. If necessary, take lipid-lowering drugs.

　To have good food habits, an individual should practice on the base of the standard diet therapy, step by step.

REVIEW QUESTIONS

I Select the correct definition for each term.
 1. cerebrovascular disease   2. low-density lipoprotein cholesterol
 3. atherosclerosis   4. unsaturated fatty acid   5. hypercholesterolemia
   a) A disease of the arteries characterized by irregularly distributed lipid deposits in their inner walls
   b) A disease relating to the blood supply to the brain, particularly with reference to pathologic changes
   c) The presence of a large amount of cholesterol in the bloodstream
   d) The so-called bad cholesterol which contains mostly lipid and few proteinous elements
   e) A carboxylic acid, the carbon chain with double or triple bonds and therefore can incorporate additional hydrogen atoms

II Write the appropriate term on the line.
 1. Hyperlipidemia is an abnormal excess of any or all fatty substances typically _____, and triacylglycerol.
 2. Hyperlipidemia is caused in part from being overweight and consuming a diet high in _____ fats and cholesterol.
 3. In China and Japan, _____ disease is less common than it is in countries such as the United States.
 4. The total cholesterol level is a general guide to the risk of _____ with assessment of diabetes, hypertension and obesity.
 5. The treatment for hyperlipidemia is to change their life style, that is, to keep an appropriate _____, stop smoking, and increase physical activity.

III Write T for true, F for false on the line.
 1._____ Neither low density lipoprotein nor high density lipoprotein has no relation to hyperlipidemia.
 2._____ The fundamental factors of hyperlipidemia have close relation with family or its members.
 3._____ The risk of developing atherosclerosis increases as cholesterol level decreases.
 4._____ Levels of LDL and HDL cholesterol, triacylglycerol are measured after fasting at least 12 hours before the blood sample is taken.
 5._____ The Japan Atherosclerosis Society has fixed the standard diet therapy for prevention of atherosclerotic cardiovascular diseases since 2007.

2. Diabetes Mellitus　糖尿病

　糖尿病は，インスリン分泌異常に起因する慢性代謝疾患である．病因は遺伝的因子と環境的因子とされているが，大きく1型糖尿病（免疫疾患）と2型糖尿病（インスリン分泌不足か抵抗性）に分類される．身体のエネルギー源であるブドウ糖（グルコース）をコントロールするインスリンの量が不足し作用できなくなると，血中に糖が蓄積し，持続的に高血糖状態となる．その結果，口渇，多尿，体重減少，倦怠感などの症状が現れ，血糖コントロールを放置すると神経障害，網膜症，腎症などの合併症を発症する．また動脈硬化の原因となり，心筋梗塞や脳梗塞が起きる．重篤の状態では昏睡状態から死に至るケースも多い．特に治療には確実な医学的治療法はなく，肥満が最大のポイントであることから，食事療法が第一である．あわせて適度の運動と，タイプに合ったインスリンや経口血糖下降剤投与，透析がなされる．日本では食事や運動の生活習慣が関連する2型糖尿病が95％を占めるが，さらに増加しつつあり，重要な健康問題となっている．

KEY WORDS

Select the Japanese term most appropriate for each English term.
1. complication   2. fast eating   3. fasting plasma glucose test
4. genotypes   5. hemoglobin A1c   6. maturity onset diabetes
7. polyuria   8. insulin injection   9. insulin dependent diabetes
10. type 2 diabetes mellitus
a. ヘモグロビンA1c   b. 空腹時血糖テスト   c. 多尿   d. 合併症
e. 2型糖尿病   f. 成人発症型糖尿病   g. インスリン依存型糖尿病
h. 遺伝子型   i. 早食い   j. インスリン注射

[DESCRIPTION]

　Diabetes mellitus is a chronic carbohydrate metabolic disorder caused by insufficient secretion of insulin or inadequate response of the body cells to this hormone in the body's cells. Prolonged hyperglycemia (accumulation of glucose in the blood) leads to the classical symptoms of polyuria, polydipsia and polyphagia. It also develops to be a risk factor of some complications. The incorrect fat-glucose mixture in the tissue will cause incomplete combustion of the fat which, if unchecked, sometimes results in death.

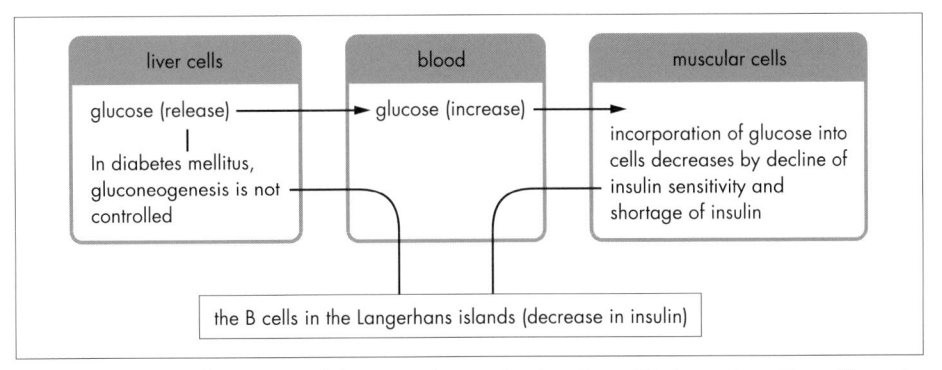

```
┌─────────────────────────────────────────────────────────────────┐
│  ┌──────────────┐    ┌──────────────┐    ┌──────────────────┐  │
│  │  liver cells │    │    blood     │    │  muscular cells  │  │
│  ├──────────────┤    ├──────────────┤    ├──────────────────┤  │
│  │ glucose (release)─→ glucose (increase)→ incorporation of  │  │
│  │      │       │    │              │    │ glucose into     │  │
│  │ In diabetes  │    │              │    │ cells decreases  │  │
│  │ mellitus,    │────┤              │    │ by decline of    │  │
│  │ gluconeogenesis│  │              │    │ insulin sensitivity│ │
│  │ is not       │    │              │    │ and shortage of  │  │
│  │ controlled   │    │              │    │ insulin          │  │
│  └──────────────┘    └──────────────┘    └──────────────────┘  │
│                            ↑                    ↑               │
│              ┌─────────────┴────────────────────┴───────┐      │
│              │ the B cells in the Langerhans islands    │      │
│              │ (decrease in insulin)                    │      │
│              └──────────────────────────────────────────┘      │
└─────────────────────────────────────────────────────────────────┘
```

Figure 21 Mechanism of hyperglycemia by insufficient insulin effect in diabetes mellitus（糖尿病におけるインスリン作用不足による高血糖のメカニズム）

[ETIOLOGY]

The cause of diabetes depends on the type. Type 1 diabetes is partly inherited and then triggered by certain infections, with some evidence pointing at the *Coxsackie B4 virus*. There is a genetic element in individual susceptibility to some of these triggers which has been traced to particular HLA genotypes (i.e. the genetic "self" identifiers relied upon by the immune system). However, even in those who have inherited the susceptibility, type 1 diabetes mellitus seems to require an environmental trigger. Type 2 diabetes is due primarily to lifestyle.

[CLASSFICATION]

There are two main types and two other types of diabetes:
1) Type 1 diabetes (insulin-dependent diabetes, juvenile diabetes) results from the full shortage of insulin secreted by the B cells in the Langerhans islands. As fat cannot be adequately burned, the disease will be fatal, if unchecked and treated, with the clinical condition of ketoacidosis.

   In Japan, the incidence of this form is 10-15 per 100,000 population, which is much lower than in Western countries.
2) Type 2 diabetes (non-insulin-dependent diabetes mellitus, maturity onset diabetes) results from relative loss of insulin. This more common form has two dominant abnormalities: reduced insulin sensitivity (insulin resistance), and decreased insulin secretion in

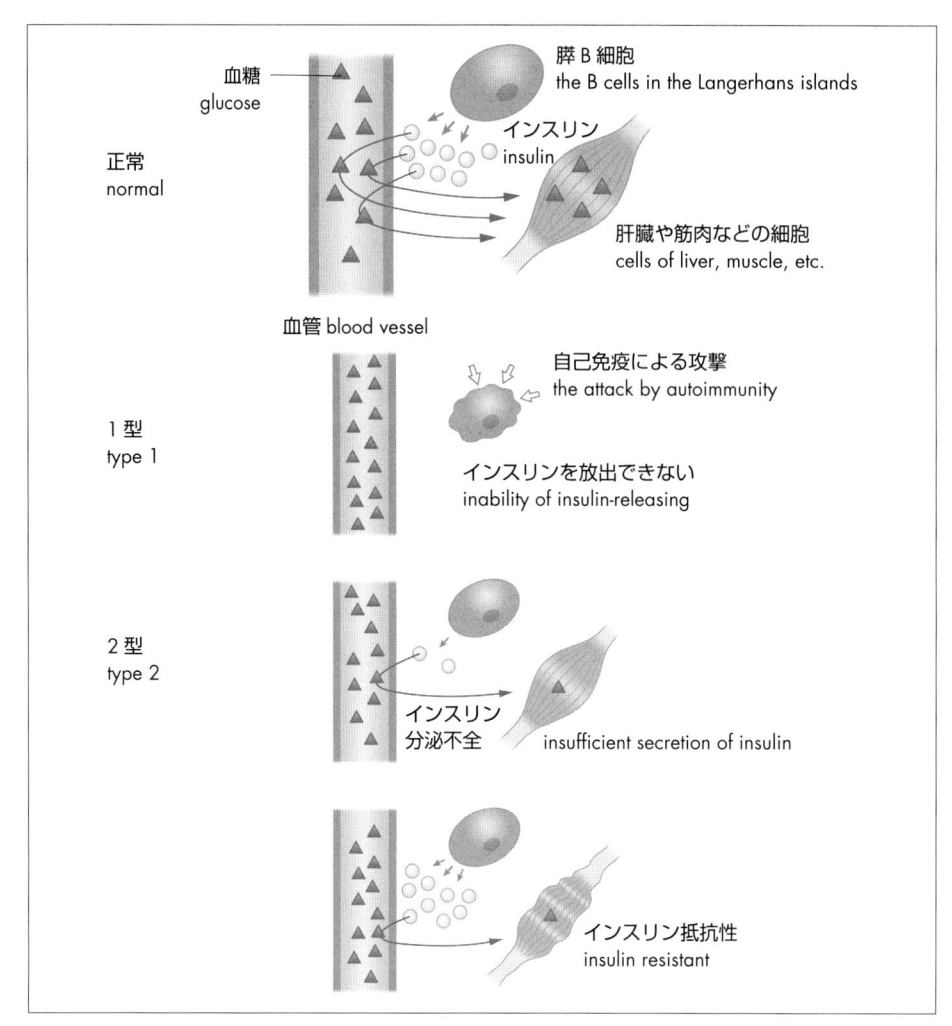

Figure 22 Diabetes mellitus（糖尿病）

 the B cells in the Langerhans islands, resulting in hyperglycemia.
  In Japan, the incidence of this form accounts for 95% of the patients with diabetes.
3) Other specific types of diabetes refers to congenital diabetes identified as genetic factor (e.g. the insulin gene factor, glucokinase gene), and other dysfunctions with pancreatic dysfunctions caused by drugs, and infections.
4) Gestational diabetes can be found in women during pregnancy which often disappears after delivery but sometimes develops into type 2 diabetes in later years.

gestational diabetes：妊娠糖尿病（GDM）.

[SIGNS and SYMPTOMS]

The classic symptoms of most cases of diabetes mellitus are those mentioned in the description above and in the following table. Some differences between Type 1 and Type 2 are also shown in the table below.

[DIAGNOSIS]

The individual's presenting symptoms may suggest a diagnosis of diabetes mellitus. A fasting plasma glucose test and hemoglobin A1c (HbA1c) level are the preferred way to diagnose diabetes.

[TREATMENT]

A combination of diet, insulin, and exercise is used to treat most forms of diabetes mellitus. Individuals with type 1 diabetes typically need to follow a consistent dietary pattern that is closely linked to the

Table 7　Overview of the most significant symptoms of diabetes（糖尿病の症状）

Feature	type 1 diabetes mellitus	type 2 diabetes mellitus
Onset	sudden	gradual
Prevalence	−5%	95%−
Age at onset	mostly in youth	mostly in adults
Ketoacidosis	common	rare
Body Physique	often thin	often obese (30%−40%)
Concordance with family history (inherited)	often (−) but not clear	often (+) often and strong
Correlation with HLA	(+)	(−)
Virus infection	(+)	(−)
Autoantibodies	(+)	(−)
Insulin secretion	extremely decreased or absent	slightly or medium decrease
Insulin therapy	essential	generally unessential or rarely essential

Table 8　Diabetes diagnostic criteria（糖尿病の診断基準）

Condition	2 hour glucose*	Fasting plasma glucose	HbA1c
Normal	<140 mg/dL	<110 mg/dL	
Diabetes mellitus	≧200 mg/dL	≧126 mg/dL	≧6.5%
Border line	Not belong to diabetic or normal type		

＊75 g oral glucose tolerance test (75 g OGTT)

insulin injection. A consistent routine of exercise will lessen the need for insulin. Those with type 2 diabetes usually require a diet that restricts their energy intake. Diet therapy alone may be all that is necessary to control their symptoms. If not, hypoglycemic drugs may be prescribed. These drugs act to stimulate insulin production or make body cells more sensitive to insulin. In some instances, those with type 2 diabetes also may require injected insulin.

1) Medications

a) Anti-diabetic medication

Metformin hydrochloride is generally recommended as a first line treatment for type 2 diabetes as there is good evidence that it decreases mortality.

Routine use of aspirin however has not been found to improve outcomes in uncomplicated diabetes.

b) Insulin therapy

Type 1 diabetes is typically treated with a combination of regular and NPH (neutral protamine hagedorn) insulin or synthetic insulin analogs. When insulin is used in type 2 diabetes, a long-acting formulation is usually added initially, while continuing oral medications. Doses of insulin are then increased for effect.

2) Dietary management

The standard diet management is:

a) Establishment of regular dietary habits

Dietary habits such as skipping a meal, joint eating, rapid eating, eating at midnight, frequent eating out, and too much eating of favorite foods should be refrained from because they lead to derangement of the control of blood sugar.

b) Adequate energy intake

Adequate energy intake should be determined to keep standard body weight. A day's intake energy is temporarily determined by multiplying 22-40 kcal/kg by standard body weight, taking into consideration for one's age, sex, the level physical activity and a built. For example, the plan of consuming energy intake needs to be reexamined as their lifestyle in hospital and after discharge changes greatly.

c) Diets with good balanced nutrition

Table 9 Diet therapy based on nutrients （栄養素別食事療法）

nutrient	daily diet therapy
energy requirement by standard body weight	light work : 25–30 kcal/kg medium work : 30–35 kcal/kg hard work : 35– kcal/kg
protein	* Attention is paid to excessive intake so as to prevent from nephropathy. * Standard protein intake is about 1 g/kg. * Protein intake is more restricted according to the level of nephropathy. (1.0–1.2 g/kg)
lipid	* Excessive lipid intake deranges blood glycemic control and facilitates arteriosclerosis. * The standard energy-lipid ratio is 20%–25%. * Cutting down on intake of animal saturated fatty acid but recommending to take multivalent unsaturated fatty acid including fishes.
carbohydrate	* As low molecular sucrose causes hyperglycemia because of its easy absorption, macromolecular starch is recommended. * Carbohydrates of which the energy ratio is almost 50–60% is the main energy source
vitamin/mineral	* Keeping Dietary Reference Intakes (DRIs) level, because these intakes are apt to decrease with a decrease energy intake. Especially fat-soluble vitamins are supposed to decrease with fatty intake decreasing. (Calcium and iron also tend to be lacking.)
salt	Salt intake should be cut down, because consuming of other seasoning also increases at the same time with salt intake increasing. ～ 10 g/day

It has recently been pointed out that intake of lipids, especially animal lipids or refined foods should be limited, and vitamin, mineral or dietary fiber intake tends to be insufficient in the Western diet. The dietary therapy for diabetes is intended for prevention of complications, such as microangiopathy and arteriosclerosis. Therefore, not only appropriate energy intake but efforts to ensure good balanced nutrition including three major nutrients, vitamin, mineral and dietary fiber of all sorts is also recommended for keeping healthy mind and body.

three major nutrients : protein, lipid, cabohydrate.

REVIEW QUESTIONS

I Select the correct definition for each term.
   1. diabetes mellitus   2. complication   3. polyuria
   4. fasting plasma glucose   5. insulin
   a) A secondary disease or condition that makes a previous one more confused or difficult
   b) A metabolic disorder in which the body cannot control sugar absorption because the pancreas does not produce enough insulin
   c) A test for blood levels of the substance measured when the patient has not eaten for a giving duration, generally in the morning
   d) A hormone secreted by B cells in the Langerhans islands which regulates carbohydrate and fat metabolism in the body
   e) Production of abnormally large volumes of dilute urine

II Write the appropriate term on the line.
   1. Diabetes mellitus is a chronic carbohydrate _____ caused by insufficient secretion of insulin.
   2. Type 2 diabetes mellitus is due primarily to _____ factors and _____.
   3. In Japan, the incidence of type 2 diabetes mellitus accounts for _____ of the patients with diabetes.
   4. Those with type 2 diabetes mellitus usually require a diet that restricts their _____.
   5. Efforts to take good balanced nutrition including three major nutrients, _____, _____ and _____ of all sorts is also recommended.

III Write T for true, F for false on the line.
   1. ____ An unbalanced fat-glucose mixture in the tissue will cause incomplete combustion of the fat which, if unchecked, sometimes results in death.
   2. ____ Type 1 diabetes is partly acquired and Type 2 diabetes mellitus is primarily inherited.
   3. ____ Type 2 diabetes mellitus results from the relative shortage of insulin secreted by the B cells within the Langerhans islands.
   4. ____ Individuals with type 1 diabetes only need injections of insulin.
   5. ____ Diet therapy may be all that is necessary to control symptoms for people with type 2 diabetes.

Unit 9
Nutritional Diseases and Disorders
栄養疾患

Introduction to Malnutrition

What is malnutrition?

Malnutrition generally refers to poor nutritional conditions that includes either undernutrition and overnutrition. The former often results from taking insufficient diet or improper specific dietary components, and the latter by excess or imbalanced consumption of nutrients.

Undernutrition, especially protein-energy malnutrition (PEM), is more common in developing countries, where many children are not able to take adequate energy and protein because of food shortage. In affluent societies, on the contrary, people tend to be in either undernutrition or overnutrition because of their taking unbalanced diet, for example, fast food, empty calorie foods or luxurious but unhealthy diet.

In Japan, with the advent of an aged society, malnutrition is a current health problem of the elderly people especially in long-term nursing care homes as well as in hospitals where they are in the their bed-ridden lives and patients cannot fully utilize the food. They sometimes suffer from the severity of primary diseases or infectious or not-infectious diseases. To improve their conditions, not only nutritionists but physicians, dentists, nurses, pharmacists, and social workers are expected to take part in the planning of their diet.

long-term nursing care home：長期高齢者介護福祉施設.

1. Protein-energy Malnutrition
たんぱく質・エネルギー栄養障害

　たんぱく質・エネルギー栄養障害は，たんぱく質およびエネルギーの欠乏によって生じる栄養不良の状態をいう．特にカシオコア（クワシオルコル）とマラスムス，その中間の重篤なタイプの中間型重症たんぱく質・エネルギー栄養障害症候群は，干ばつや不足紛争の多発する開発途上国において食糧危機，母体の栄養不良などによって起きる，死亡率の高い重症型の栄養障害である．しかし，豊かな文明国家においてもたんぱく質・エネルギー障害は例外ではなく，格差社会においては貧しい家庭に見られ社会的健康問題のひとつとされている．日本においても同様であり，拒食症・過食症のような心理的要因による摂食障害，後天性免疫不全症候群（AIDS）のような現代特有の病気，さまざま習慣病患者の増加，高齢者の増加に伴ってたんぱく質・エネルギー障害は重要な健康問題となっている．特に高齢者を含む入院や施設入居における軽度から重篤な患者に対して，さらにその予備軍に対する適切な栄養摂取・補給の対策が急がれている．

KEY WORDS

Select the Japanese term most appropriate for each English term.
1. dosage   2. immobilization   3. ingestion   4. kwashiorkor
5. marasmus   6. nitrogen   7. parenteral alimentation
8. muscle atrophy   9. sarcopenia   10. undernutrition
a. 筋量減少症   b. マラスムス（消耗症）   c. 窒素   d. 投与   e. 不動
f. クワシオルコル（食事性たんぱく質欠乏症候群）   g. 筋萎縮
h. 経口摂取   i. 非経口的栄養法   j. 栄養不足

[DESCRIPTION]

　There are two main types of protein-energy malnutrition (PEM): kwashiorkor caused by deficient protein in the food, and marasmus, a state of severe undernourishment, resulted from insufficient intake of food. These ill conditions mostly occur in children and prenatal babies both in the developing countries.

　In the affluent society, some factors such as fad diets, ignorance of the nutritional diets and food allergy (commonly milk and egg allergy) also develop PEM in children. At the same time, PEM results from such impairments as chronic diseases, cancer, acquired immunodeficiency syndrome (AIDS) and psychological eating disorders (e.g. anorexia and bulimia nervosa). Recently in Japan, PEM has become a target health problem of the aged people who easily develop malnutrition by decreasing intake of the staple food and side dishes during their aging process.

[ETIOLOGY]

As mentioned above, PEM results from deficiency of protein and energy in the diet intake, and there are some differences among the types of the PEM as follows.

a) Kwashiorkor: This condition describes the dangerous form of protein deficiency, typically affecting young children in the developing countries. There, when the second baby is born, the first-born child's food is changed from breast-feeding to a food (corn) which is rich with carbohydrate but not protein.

b) Marasmus: This severe debilitating condition is caused by total deficiency in energy intake commonly in children.

c) Marasmic Kwashiorkor: The most severe form of malnutrition due to both ill-conditions of protein deficiency (kwashiorkor) and energy deficiency (marasmus).

d) Moderate and unspecified PEM: This is moderate condition including general PEM.

e) PEM in hospitalized patients: PEM including general malnutrition can be caused not only by such factors as diarrhea, fever, hemorrhage, glycosuria, kidney disease, and cancer, but others including injuries, burn injury, infection and surgery and some medications.

f) PEM in the elderly: Aging process and changes of their life style influence the elderly both in their way of eating or inadequate dietary intake and their diseases. Chewing problem or swallowing difficulties leads to decreased appetite. Moreover psychological factors such as sorrow from parting their spouses or depression by anxiety for their aging also triggers their loss of appetite, as well as

---

Marasmic Kwashiokor：severe PEM-unqualified. 中間型重症たんぱく質・エネルギー栄養障害症候群.
Moderate and unspecified PEM：中等度たんぱく質・栄養障害症候群.

decline in their energy and well-being.

[SIGNS and SYMPTOMS]

a) Kwashiorkor: acute characteristic symptoms are incomplete development, generalized edema, distended abdomen with progressive protein deficiency. Muscle atrophy, fatty liver, skin depigmentation, thinning hair, anemia, diarrhea, neurological disorder also occur at the same time.

b) Marasmus: A marked underweight (less than 60% of a child with healthy body) leads to loss of subcutaneous fat and muscle atrophy.

c) Marasmic Kwashiokor: both symptoms of kwashiokor and marasmus are revealed.

d) Moderate and unspecified PEM: moderate symptoms including general malnutrition are developed.

e) PEM in hospitalized patients: Patients have difficulty in chewing, swallowing and digesting food, pain, nausea, and lack of appetite.

f) PEM in the elderly: Coupled with sarcopenia, the muscle function, and immobility in their daily lives are lost. Then, skeletal disorders, hypertension, atherosclerosis, and metabolic disorders follow.

[DIAGNOSIS]

When one of indexes in the following is applicable, an individual is diagnosed as PEM and then, need to have diet therapy.

＊Nitrogen balance: continuance of the negative value more than a week

＊Percentage of the standard body weight: less than 80%

＊Density of albumin: less than 3.0 g/dL

＊Density of transferrin: less than 200 mg/dL

＊Total number of lymphocyte: less than 1,000/μL

＊Tuberculin reaction: less than 5 mm

skin depigmentation：色素脱失.　subcutaneous：皮下脂肪.

[TREATMENT]

Nutritional treatment carries out on the basis of direct assessment by clinical test, physical measurement and indirect assessment by diet inspection.

The nutritional standard is shown in 1), and matters to require attention is in 2) below.

1) The nutritional standard

Energy intake

a) The level is decided on the careful observation of energy consumption of the patient.

b) 500 kcal per day and 250 kcal is added every day (the utmost adding carbohydrate is 60 g per day.)

Protein

a) Quantity of protein to maintain nitrogen balance: 1.0 g/kg/day

b) During a period of growth: more than 1.5 g/kg/day

c) In the case of nutritional disorder: 1.5–2.0 g/kg/day

2) Matters to be paid attention

a) Basic nutrition supply: By taking nutrition in diet. Parenteral alimentation is for a special case.

b) Nutrition: Supplement without harmful side effects and suitable quantity for the patient

c) Nutrition for the patient with severe PEM: Gradual supply not to cause complications of heart, blood vessels or metabolism. As the patient with severe PEM whose body weight is less than 50% of standard body weight tends to have fatty liver, high aspartate aminotransferase (AST) or alanine transaminase (ALT), dosage of nutrition should be carefully observed.

d) Protein intake: If any abnormal change in the blood serum urea nitrogen (BUN) density is found, dosage of protein must be reduced.

e) Education of nutrition: Patients are educated about nutrient supply and how to eat diets that patients cook themselves.

f) Malnutrition in the elderly: Both adequate nutrition supply and independent eating without anyone's help.

Let's take a break.

今回が最後のbreakです．そこで趣向を変えて早口言葉（a tongue twister）を練習しましょう．

The sixth sick sheik's sixth sheep's sick.
6番目の長老が飼っている6番目の羊が病気です．

舌を噛みそうですが's'と'she'の発音を明確にすることが大切．
ところで，日本語でも「病気」「疾病」「疾患」「障害」とあるように，英語でも病気の状態を表すものがいくつかあり，以下のように内容がいくぶん異なります．

disease：病気・疾患・疾病
  1) 身体の構造・器官などに断絶が見られるか，停止，障害がある場合
  2) 病因物質をもち，明らかな兆候や症候群がある．
disorder：障害・疾患
  1) 遺伝性，外因性要因による異常な機能的，器質的変化
  2) 軽い病気，心身の不調・異常・障害
illness：特定の病気，精神病（mental illness）
  sickness：不健康，吐き気，不調
  syndrome：症候群．複数の症状・兆候の組み合わせによって形成される病態．
      原因が多岐にわたる場合もある．

ほかにailment, morbus, trouble, disturbanceもあります．"Oh, I got sick and can't go on anymore."という声が聴こえてきます．

時には元気を出すために音楽を聴きましょうか？ 聴覚障害者，ベートーベンの「熱情（Passion）」でもいかがですか？ そういえば，passionのpassio-も，病理学pathologyのpatho-も，患者patientのpati-もすべて「苦しむ」という意味です．

clinical（＝bedside）nutritionistの前にいるのは，disease（easeをdisされた状態）を患うpatientであり，co-medical（co-共に＋medic医療の・医師＋-alに関する），NST（nutrition support team：栄養サポートチーム）の中心にいるのは，patientのはずですね．

REVIEW QUESTIONS

I Select the correct definition for each term.
  1. parenteral alimentation   2. dosage   3. ingestion
  4. sarcopenia   5. muscle atrophy
   a) An amount, frequency, and number of medicine prescribed by a doctor
   b) Introduction of nutrition, food, drink by swallowing into the stomach
   c) Providing the body with nutrition elsewhere in the body by the form of injection
   d) Progress reduction of muscle tissue as a natural part of the aging process
   e) The condition of losing flesh, muscle strength, etc. in part of the body because of immobility or other causes

II Write the appropriate term on the line.
  1. There are two main types of protein-energy malnutrition: _____ and _____.
  2. In Japan, the elderly people in home or in hospital tend to have PEM because of decreasing intake of the _____ and _____.
  3. For the elderly, changes in body composition, functional _____ in organs and diseases can be causes of decreased appetite.
  4. Coupled with _____ with loss of muscle function, being underweight brings about immobilization for the elderly.
  5. As the patient with severe PEM whose body weight is less than 50% of _____, _____ of nutrition should be carefully observed.

III Write T for true, F for false on the line.
  1. ____ Protein-energy malnutrition includes only protein deficiency in the diet.
  2. ____ People in Japan do not have any health problem of PEM as in the developing countries.
  3. ____ The cause of PEM in the elderly includes psychological depression or anxiety of their aging process.
  4. ____ The elderly in the facilities or hospital tend to fall into a stay into a life in bed because of PEM.
  5. ____ To supply nutrition, parenteral alimentation is more effective for the nutrient supply the patient with PEM than ingestion.

2. Dysphagia (Swallowing Disorder)
嚥下障害

　嚥下障害とは，食物や水分を口腔から食道，胃へと送りこむ嚥下の過程において，飲みこみにくい，むせる，のどにつまる症状をいう．一般的には，脳・脊髄神経，筋肉，舌・咽頭・喉頭がん，あるいは恐食症など心理的な疾患，また，加齢に伴う症状のひとつであるが，独立した障害として見なされる場合もある．食物の摂取・嚥下は，身体的生命活動を可能にする呼吸や栄養吸収に不可欠な活動であることは言うまでもない．さらに，食事は生活における楽しみでもあり，食卓を共にすることによってより深いコミュニケーションを導く重要な意味をもつ．また食する人々が住む地域，国の個性を表す文化的共有物でもある．その障害は，人の生命に危険な状態を引き起こすばかりでなく，食を巡るさまざまな楽しみから遠ざけてしまう．このような意味で管理栄養士は他の医療関係者とともに嚥下障害に適切に対処するために，症状の原因ばかりでなく患者のQOLを意識した食事スタイルを確立することが求められている．

KEY WORDS

Select the Japanese term most appropriate for each English term.
1. accidental swallowing (pulmonary aspiration)
2. cerebrovascular accident   3. choking   4. esophageal dysphagia
5. oropharyngeal dysphagia   6. percutaneous endoscopic gastrostomy
7. repeated saliva swallowing test   8. tube feeding
9. videoendoscopic examination
10. videofluorographic examination
a. 嚥下造影検査   b. 嚥下内視鏡検査   c. 経管栄養法
d. 経皮的内視鏡下胃瘻造設術   e. 口腔咽頭嚥下障害   f. 誤嚥
g. 食道性嚥下障害   h. 脳血管障害   i. 反復唾液嚥下テスト   j. むせること

[DESCRIPTION]

　Dysphagia generally refers to difficulty swallowing or choking sensation when solid food or liquid passes from the oral cavity to the esophagus, then to the stomach. The process is classified into two major types: oropharyngeal dysphagia (trouble with moving food from the mouth to the upper esophagus) and esophageal dysphagia

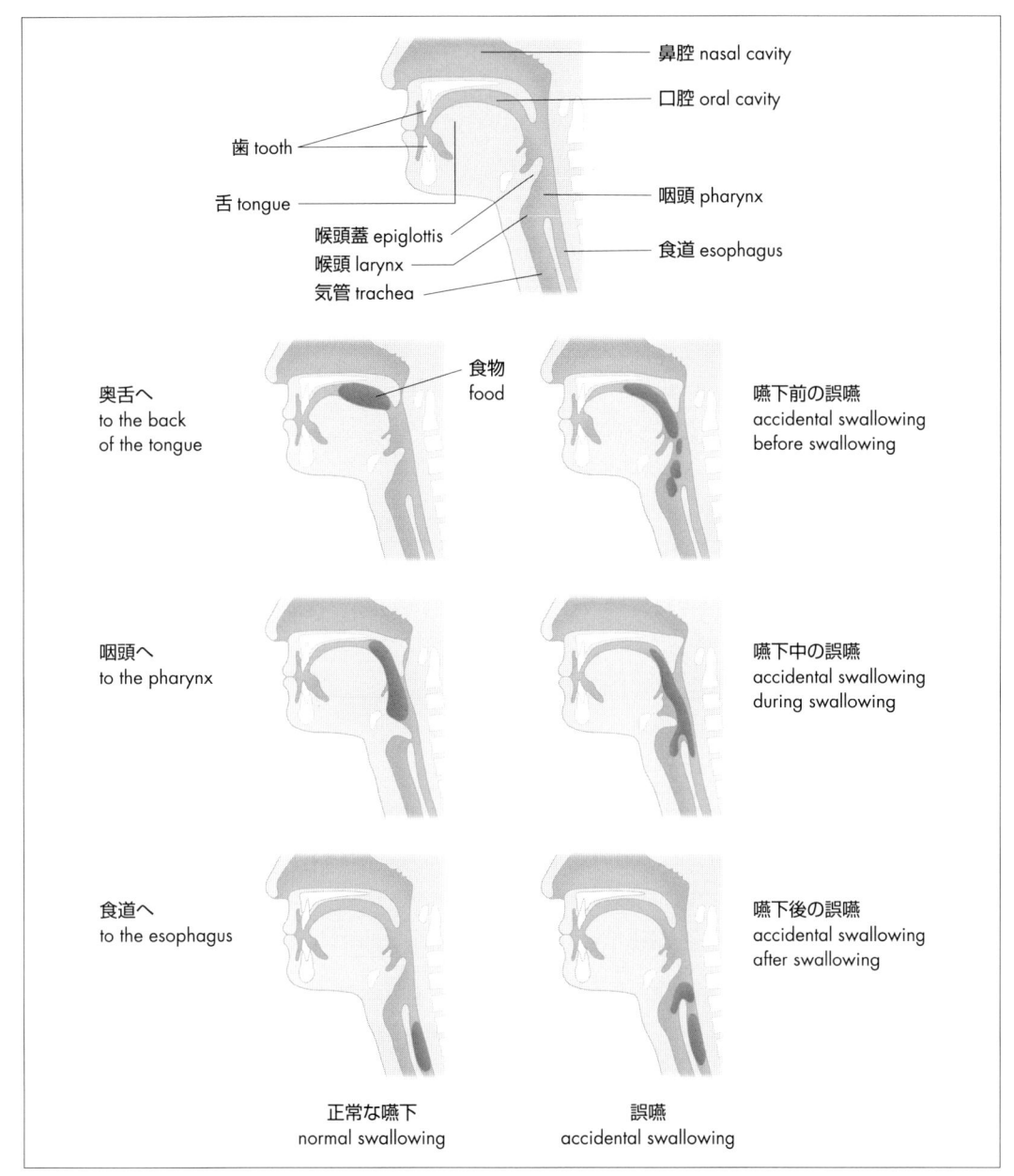

Figure 23 Normal swallowing and accidental swallowing（嚥下と誤嚥）

(through the esophagus to the stomach). The latter is the most common type of dysphagia.

These disorders quite often occur among the elderly. However, they can also occur in people of all ages who have congenital abnormalities, damage of the organ and/or medical conditions. For example, people who have had stroke, or patients who are admitted to hospitals or care facilities can also suffer from dysphagia.

[ETIOLOGY]

Dysphagia is a symptom with many different causes. Swallowing food involves intricate cooperation between cerebral nerves and many muscles of the oral organs and esophagus, so, dysphagia may be related to consciousness disturbance. Disorders leading to dysphagia are roughly into the following 3 categories.

1) Organic disorders

Inflammation of the organs inside the mouth, around the pharynx, and esophagus or injuries after operation (e.g. lingual cancer, pharyngeal cancer) may lead to organic dysphagia. Organic disorders from congenital anomaly such as deformity, tortuosity and stenosis of the esophagus or hiatal hernia also cause dysphagia. Changes caused by aging can also cause dysphagia.

2) Functional disorders

Dysphagia can occur when movement of organs in the oral cavity and the pharynx are abnormal. Causes include neurological disorders such as cerebrovascular accident (stroke), head injury, Parkinson disease, amyotrophic lateral sclerosis, brain tumor, diabetic peripheral neuropathy, myasthenia gravis, muscular dystrophy or side effect of medications.

3) Psychogenic dysphagia

Even in some patients who do not have organic or functional causes, dysphagia can occur, so that lack of symptoms may not exclude an underlying disease. They sometimes complain of difficulties in eating or swallowing difficulties because of psychogenic factors such as dementia, anorexia nervosa, bulimia nervosa, psychosomatic disorder, or depression.

[SIGNS and SYMPTOMS]

Signs and symptoms in oropharyngeal dysphagia
* Spilling food from the mouth
* Impossibility or difficulty in chewing
* Increasing phlegm

myasthenia gravis：重症筋無力症.　psychosomatic disorder：心身症.

* Choking
* Regurgitating food or liquid up
* Hoarseness

Signs and symptoms in esophageal dysphagia
* Pain on swallowing
* Chest pain
* Heartburn
* Pressure sensation in the chest

Others
* Malnutrition, weight loss, dehydration, and pneumonia or asphyxia caused by accidental swallowing.
* Care is needed in cases of subclinical dysphagia.

[DIAGNOSIS]

Dysphagia is usually recognized by a careful history taking a formal dysphagia evaluation performed by a speech language pathologist.

One of the typical tests for dysphagia is the repetitive saliva swallowing test (RSST), in which the person swallows saliva or water. The so-called "gold standard" for diagnosing dysphagia is videofluorographic examination (VF) which evaluates the morphologic and functional abnormalities of various organs swallowing is found. Chest x-ray examination and pulmonary function tests are useful for detecting pulmonary disorders. Videoendoscopic examination (VE) observes the movements of the pharynx and the larynx. Blood tests can detect signs of infection or level of hydration.

[TREATMENT]

Following the result of examinations, therapeutic study is decided. If the condition of the patient is well, he/she will start direct eating training. If not, tube feeding, or surgery will be done. If possible, training of facial muscles, range of motion, swallowing and respiration and speech therapy will be tried at the same time.

repetitive saliva swallowing test (RSST)：反復唾液嚥下テスト

Dietary management

Nutritional management includes care of oral cavity, control of nutrition and liquid, and adjusting of position for eating, etc.

1) Eating training

Considering the patient's safety first, eating training should be extended step by step. Depending on the position and diet contents, some of the following matters may require attention.

a) Nutritional standard follows dietary reference intakes.
b) The diet must be safe for the patient to prevent accidental ingestion.
c) Individual preference should be respected, especially in the elderly.
d) Someone should stay with the patient when taken to prevent his/he accidental ingestion and drinking liquid.

2) Nutrient intake by nasal tube feeding and percutaneous endoscopic gastrostomy (PEG)

These feeding systems bypass or supplement dysphagia. In severe dysphagia, these methods are necessary to prevent malnutrition.

nasal tube feeding：経鼻経管栄養

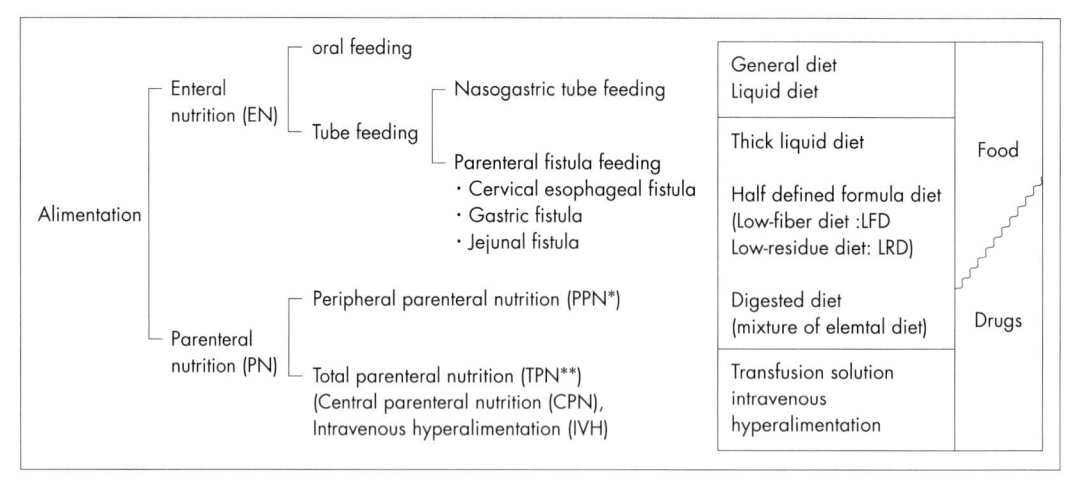

Figure 24 Alimentation（栄養補給方法）

```
                        ┌ oral feeding
         ┌ Enteral      │
         │ nutrition(EN)┤        ┌ Nasogastric tube feeding
         │              └ Tube feeding
         │                       │
         │                       └ Parenteral fistula feeding
Alimentation                        · Cervical esophageal fistula
         │                          · Gastric fistula
         │                          · Jejunal fistula
         │
         │              ┌ Peripheral parenteral nutrition (PPN*)
         └ Parenteral   │
           nutrition(PN)└ Total parenteral nutrition (TPN**)
                          (Central parenteral nutrition (CPN),
                          Intravenous hyperalimentation (IVH))
```

	Food
General diet / Liquid diet	
Thick liquid diet	
Half defined formula diet (Low-fiber diet :LFD Low-residue diet: LRD)	
Digested diet (mixture of elemtal diet)	Drugs
Transfusion solution intravenous hyperalimentation	

*日本語は，PPNの直接的訳語である「末梢非経口栄養法」とあわせて「末梢静脈栄養法」が用いられる．後者に相当するperipheral intravenous nutrition (feeding)は英語論文に用いられている．略語のPINあるいはPVNは，まだ一般的には用いられていない．

**末梢静脈栄養PPNに対し，中心静脈栄養はCPNとも説明されていたが，近年は完全静脈栄養のTPNを海外にあわせ中心静脈栄養（＝TPN）として用いており，IVHは日本においてのみ用いられている．

REVIEW QUESTIONS

I Select the correct definition for each term.
1. percutaneous endoscopic gastrostomy 2. tube feeding 3. choking
4. videofluorographic examination 5. accidental swallowing

  a) Taking food, liquid or other substances, into the larynx and lower respiratory tract by chance
  b) Having severe difficulty in breathing resulting from a foreign object in the oropharynx
  c) Procedure to create an artificial external opening into the stomach with the aid of an endoscope, most commonly to provide a means of feeding
  d) The method of administering nutrition, liquids or drugs by means of a tube inserted directly into the enteral tract
  e) The most reliable method to observe how the bolus is carried to the stomach

II Write the appropriate term on the line.
1. Dysphasia means difficulty _____ or choking sensation when solid food and liquid pass from the _____ to the esophagus.
2. Inflammation of the oral cavity, around the pharynx, and esophagus or injuries after operation, may lead to _____.
3. The so-called "gold standard" for diagnosing dysphagia is _____ by which the morphologic and functional abnormalities of various organs for swallowing are detected.
4. The diet for dysphagia must be safe for the patient to prevent _____.
5. In the case of severe _____, the patients must use the methods to prevent malnutrition.

III Write T for true, F for false on the line.
1. ____ Dysphagia generally refers to difficulty swallowing or choking when food passes to the esophagus.
2. ____ Swallowing difficulty occurs only among the elderly who are admitted to hospitals or care facilities and who also suffer from dysphagia.
3. ____ In some patients without organic or functional causes, dysphagia can occur.
4. ____ When a patient with dysphagia does direct eating training, the first matter to be paid attention for is the patient's safety.
5. ____ In the case of severe dysphagia, the patients use the methods of nutrient intake by feeding tube or through a small opening into the stomach.

Unit 10 Psychogenic Diseases and Disorders
心因性疾患

Introduction to Eating Disorders

What are eating disorders?

In Japan, eating disorders have been risen rapidly since the 1960 s. As the Ministry of Health, Labour and Welfare designated as intractable diseases, these disorders are paid attention because of difficulty to be recovered from.

Eating disorders refer not to usual keen appetite or abnormal eating behaviors, but to severe disorders based on some psychological factors such as excessive obsession concerning ideal body weight and proportions. Even if people with eating disorders have poor physical and mental health, they continue insufficient or excessive food intake.

The ICD-10 of World Health Organization (WHO) defines eating disorders under the item of Behavioural syndromes associated with physiological disturbances and physical factors.

They are grouped into mainly two types: anorexia nervosa and bulimia nervosa.

Anorexia nervosa is characterized by weight loss, induced and sustained by the patient. The disorder is often associated with a specific psychopathology whereby a dread of fatness and flabbiness of body contour persists as an intrusive overvalued idea. There is usually malnutrition of varying severity with secondary endocrine and metabolic changes and disturbances of bodily function. The symptoms include restricted dietary choice, excessive exercise,

---

since the 1960 s：日本では，テレビが普及してきた1960年代に拒食症が，コンビニエンス・ストアが増えてきた75年以降に過食症が増えてきたといわれている。　intractable diseases：中枢性摂食障害として難病に指定。　The ICD-10：International Classification of Diseases.　国際疾病分類第10版.

induced vomiting and purgation, and use of appetite suppressants and diuretics.

Bulimia nervosa is a syndrome characterized by repeated bouts of overeating and an excessive preoccupation with the control of body weight, leading to a pattern of overeating followed by vomiting or use of purgatives.

This disorder shares many psychological features with anorexia nervosa, including an overconcern with body shape and weight. Repeated vomiting is likely to give rise to disturbances of body electrolytes and physical complications. There is often, but not always, a history of an earlier episode of anorexia nervosa, the interval ranging from a few months to several years.

Eating disorders occur more among women, especially younger women, than among men, however, they affect boys, men, and older women up to menopause.

1. Anorexia Nervosa　神経性食欲不振症

　神経性食欲不振症は，摂食障害のひとつ．器質的あるいは特定の疾患がなく，節食，拒食，不食，激しい運動などによって適正体重の20％以上痩せた状態（典型的には25％以上，欧米では15％以上）．発症が30歳以下の主として女性，特に思春期前後の女性に見られる食行動の異常である．女性らしさあるいは成熟嫌悪に基づくやせ願望が強く，少しの体重増加でも極端に恐怖を覚え，醜くなったと思いこむ．そのために食事量が減少し，栄養の偏り，低栄養，便秘，貧血，低体重，女性ホルモン分泌不足，無月経などの症状が起きる．極度の低血糖が続くと意識障害，脳委縮などの障害が生じる．早期治療によって早く回復することもあるが，心身症外来や精神保健センターなどで家族を含む治療と指導が必要とされる．

KEY WORDS

Select the Japanese term most appropriate for each English term.
1. amenorrhea　2. anemia　3. deficiency　4. food refusal
5. malnutrition　6. psychogenic eating disorder
7. psychiatric disorder　8. psychotherapy　9. starvation　10. The DSM
a. 栄養不良　b. 拒食　c. 飢餓　d. 欠乏症　e. 心因性摂食障害
f. 精神障害　g. 精神療法　h. 精神障害の診断と統計の手引き
i. 無月経　j. 貧血

[DESCRIPTION]

　Anorexia nervosa is a complex psychogenic eating disorder. The key feature is usually self-imposed starvation and an irrational fear of gaining weight, even when the individual is already emaciated. It is also marked by weight loss, clinical evidence of semistarvation, amenorrhea, and an alteration in body image. In Japan as in other developed countries, this disorder is becoming a major health problem, especially in women in their teen and twenties who tend to regard a slim body as their ideal image.

[ETIOLOGY]

　The cause of anorexia nervosa is not known, although most health professionals believe it is essentially a psychiatric disorder. Some theorists believe the refusal to eat is a subconscious effort for slimness with beauty, playing some role in provoking the disorder. A patient's socioeconomic status, family background, and cultural conditioning may be predisposing factors in the development of the condition.

[SIGNS and SYMPTOMS]

A loss of 20% or more of original body weight, in the absence of any detectable underlying medical disorder, may suggest a diagnosis of anorexia nervosa. Evidence of food refusal, vomiting, and excessive exercise also suggest the diagnosis. In severe cases, a host of secondary symptoms may appear as a result of metabolic and hormonal disturbances (amenorrhea) resulting from malnutrition. The affected individual also may tend to deny feelings of hunger and will typically claim to be overweight despite physical evidence to the contrary.

[DIAGNOSIS]

Worldwide diagnosing criteria depend on The DSM-IV, a doctors' manual for psychiatric diseases published by American Psychiatric Association. In Japan, careful interpretation of clinical data is necessary to rule out other disorders that cause physical wasting. No specific diagnostic test exists for anorexia nervosa, but blood testing may reveal associated nutritional anemia and vitamin or mineral deficiencies.

[TREATMENT]

Medical treatment of anorexia nervosa is aimed at reversing the effects of malnutrition and controlling the individual compulsion to binge eating. Aggressive medical management, nutritional counseling, and individual and family psychotherapy are

---

20% or more of original body weight：厚生労働省特定疾患診断基準．1) 標準体重の－20％，2) 不食，大食，隠れ食いなどの食行動の異常，3) 体重・体形への認識の歪み，4) 発症年齢30歳以下，5) 無月経，6) 器質的疾患がない．　DSM-IV：Diagnostic and Statistical Manual of Mental Disorders．米国精神医学会作成の精神疾患の診断・統計マニュアル．DSM-I (1952) 以来版を重ねている．また，ICD-10との統合も検討されている．2000年の診断基準は，1) 標準体重の15％，2) 体重減少時にも，体重増加に恐怖心をもつ，3) 標準体重に満たない時も体重過多と感じる，4) 3周期以上の無月経である．なお，2013年予定のDSM-Vでは4) の条件がなくなっている．

recommended.

Referring the patient and family members to the local and welfare mental health center, the public health center, and psychological counselor's office attached to a university for additional information and support can be beneficial. Hospitalization may be required in the event of severe weight loss and malnutrition.

1) Dietary management

The goal of dietary management is to let the patient have a regular good balanced diet. However, they may be anxious about eating so they should be allowed to eat their favorite foods or foods easy to eat to maintain proper energy intake. It is necessary to give nutritional guidance according to their acceptable weight with understanding of their fear for obesity. Foods on the market on which energy values shown or high energy enteral nutrients are useful for nutritional therapy. In addition, it may be necessary to stay with the individual during and after meals and to give rewards for their efforts.

The standard of nutrition is as follows:

a) In order to prevent and improve protein-energy malnutrition (PEM), proper energy requirement as well as protein requirement should be taken.

b) The patient's energy intake should correspond to his/her energy expenditure.

c) The energy intake is begun from approximately 500 kcal/day and is added 250 kcal every day.

d) In order to keep nitrogen balance, protein (1.0 g/kg/day) is needed. During a period of growth, 1.5 g/kg/day and in the state of malnutrition: 1.5–2.0 g/kg/day are prescribed.

protein-energy malnutrition：厚生労働省は，最近，高齢者の低栄養の表現としてPEMを用いているが，本来はたんぱく質・エネルギー栄養障害． requirement：必要量． intake：摂取量．

REVIEW QUESTIONS

I Select the correct definition for each term.
 1. malnutrition   2. protein-energy malnutrition
 3. psychogenic eating disorder   4. psychiatric disorder   5. vomitting
   a) To eject food from stomach back out through the mouth
   b) A poor condition of health caused by a lack of food, a lack of the right type of food, imperfect absorption of food material or over eating
   c) A poor health condition as a result of an deficient intake of protein and energy.
   d) Abnormal eating habits that may involve either insufficient or excessive food intake due to individual's psychological condition
   e) Disruption of normal physical or mental functions relating to mental illness or its treatment

II Write the appropriate term on the line.
 1. Anorexia nervosa is a complex _____ eating disorder.
 2. The cause of anorexia nervosa is not known, although most health professionals believe it is essentially a _____ disorder.
 3. Evidence of _____, vomiting, and excessive exercise also suggest the diagnosis.
 4. No specific diagnostic test exists for anorexia nervosa, but blood testing may reveal associated nutritional _____ and vitamin or mineral _____.
 5. In order to prevent _____, proper energy requirement as well as protein requirement should be taken.

III Write T for true, F for flase on the line.
 1. ____ Anorexia nervosa is a psychogenic disorder in which there may be an unreasonable fear of being fat.
 2. ____ In Japan as in other developed countries, anorexia nervosa becomes a minor problem, especially women in puberty.
 3. ____ The cause of anorexia nervosa is well known, and most health professionals believe it is essentially a psychiatric disorder.
 4. ____ With positive medical management, nutritional counseling, psychotherapy for the patient and family are recommended.
 5. ____ Protein should be taken but proper energy requirement is not always needed.

2. Bulimia Nervosa　神経性大食症

　神経性大食症は，発作的に繰り返し大量の食物を食べる慢性的病態である．背景には拒食症と同様に「スリムな体型が美しい」という強い思い込みがあり，それをコントロールできないままに短時間に隠れて（多くは夜間に）食べること（むちゃ食い）が特徴である．過食のあとには体重を戻すために自発性誘発性嘔吐を行い，下剤を過度に使用する，絶食，激しい運動を行う．そのため体重は正常範囲内にあるが，下痢が日常化すれば大量のカリウムが失われ，心臓の病的症状が生じる危険性がある．また，過食後，罪悪感や自己嫌悪を覚え，うつ状態になる，さらにアルコール・薬物乱用，窃盗，自傷，自殺企図などの傾向があり，心身ともに根気強い治療が必要とされる．

KEY WORDS

Select the Japanese term most appropriate for each English term.
1. anxiety　2. binge eating　3. cardiac arrhythmia
4. depression　5. laxative abuse
6. obsessive-compulsive disorder　7. phobia　8. psychosocial factor
9. repetitive gorging　10. self-induced vomiting
a. うつ状態　b. むちゃ食い　c. 恐怖症　d. 強迫性障害
e. 下剤乱用　f. 自発性誘発性嘔吐　g. 社会心理的要因　h. 不安
i. 反復性大食　j. 不整脈

[DESCRIPTION]

　Bulimia nervosa is a psychogenic eating disorder characterized by repetitive gorging with food followed by self-induced vomiting. The condition also may involve laxative abuse, the use of diuretics, and fasting. The individual with anorexia nervosa often seems obsessed with becoming even thinner, the person with bulimia has a morbid fear of becoming fat. Other behavioral abnormalities include obsessive secrecy about the condition and sometimes food stealing. The disorder principally affects young women and may occur simultaneously with anorexia nervosa.

[ETIOLOGY]

The cause of bulimia is not known. Psychosocial factors such as family conflict, sexual abuse, and a cultural overemphasis on physical appearance may be contributing factors. There may be a struggle for a self-identity and a history of depression, anxiety, phobia, and obsessive-compulsive disorder (OCD).

[SIGNS and SYMPTOMS]

Most persons with bulimia hide the behavioral evidence of their condition, and they are often normal weight or even slightly overweight on diagnosis. They may still exhibit signs of malnutrition, however, because the binge diet of a bulimic individual is often wildly unbalanced, usually consisting of junk foods such as donuts, ice cream, and candy. Owing to the high sugar content of the binge diet and the subsequent reflux of gastric secretions also can produce a chronic sore throat.

[DIAGNOSIS]

Chronic depression low tolerance for frustration, anxiety, self-consciousness, and difficultly expressing feeling, such as anger, are common. The patient is apt to possess an exaggerated sense of guilt and have difficulty controlling impulses. Serum electrolyte studies may reveal the diagnosis. Other tests may reveal cardiac arrhythmias or evidence of renal dysfunction.

[TREATMENT]

Long-term psychotherapy is usually indicated. The bulimic person knows that the eating patterns are abnormal but is unable to control them. As with the anorexic person, noncooperation on the part of the bulimic patient generally makes treatment difficult and frustrating. Treatment concentrates on interrupting the binge-purge cycle and helping the patient regain control over eating behavior.

1) Dietary management

For nutritional therapy, total assessment together with regular physical measurement, biochemical examination, clinical examination, and checking up diets. The patient needs to be guided to eat a balanced diet regularly as equivalent for energy consumption. The guideline for patients with bulimia nervosa includes the following attention.

a) To regularly eat a suitable diet according to the patient's own hunger.
b) Not to satisfy patient's emotional hunger with food but to distinguish emotional hunger and physical one.
c) For strong hunger, add light meals two or three times a day, in addition to three balanced diets three times.
d) To refrain from eating in front of a television or in a car, but sit in front of a table with other persons.
e) To eat a warm diet slowly with chopsticks, not with hands.
f) To write down about kinds of food in a diary.
g) To get patient's mind off by having various activities in daily life for avoiding binge eating.

REVIEW QUESTIONS

I Select the correct definition for each term.
   1. laxative abuse   2. phobia   3. self-induced vomiting   4. anxiety
   5. binge eating
   a) Rapid and uncontrollable consumption of huge amounts of food and beverages and an obsessive desire to lose weight
   b) The state of feeling nervous, worried or unease about something with uncertain happening
   c) The excessive and habitual use that makes one empty bowels easily
   d) An extremely or unreasonable fear or hatred or aversion to something
   e) To persuade oneself to eject matter from the stomach back out through the mouth

II Write the appropriate term on the line.
   1. Bulimia nervosa is a psychogenic eating disorder characterized by repetitive gorging with food followed by _____.
   2. In bulimia nervosa, there may be a struggle for a self-identity and a history of depression, anxiety, phobia, and _____.
   3. Treatment concentrates to interrupting the _____ and helping the patient regain control over eating behavior.
   4. The patient needs to be guided to eat a balanced diet regularly as equivalent for _____.
   5. To get patient's mind off by having various activities in daily life for avoiding _____.

III Write T for true, F for false on the line.
   1. ____ Bulimia nervosa is a physical eating disorder characterized by eating greedily followed by vomitus brought about by oneself.
   2. ____ The cause of bulimia may be related to a patient's personal history and a cultural overemphasis on physical appearance.
   3. ____ Patients with bulimia are often normal weight or even a little overweight on diagnosis without symptoms of malnutrition.
   4. ____ Patients with bulimia tend to show psychological sides from the depths of their consciousness, though they never have physical problems.
   5. ____ Patients with bulimia are recommended to relieve their desire for eating by having various actions in daily life.

Appendix 1: Biochemical Tests of Blood/Urinalysis
血液生化学検査・尿検査

The Carbohydrates（糖質類）
(blood) glucose：BS　blood sugar（血糖）
fasting blood sugar：FBS（空腹時血糖値）
hemoglobin A1c：HbA1c（ヘモグロビンA1c）
fructosamine（フルクトサミン）
lactic acid（乳酸）

The Proteins（たんぱく質類）
total protein：TP（総たんぱく）
albumin：Alb（アルブミン）
albumin/globulin ratio：A/G
　（アルブミン／グロブリン比）
blood urea nitrogen：BUN（血中尿素窒素）
serum creatine：SCr（血清クレアチン）
creatine kinase：CK（＝creatine phosphokinase：
　CPK）（クレアチンキナーゼ）

The Lipids（脂質類）
triacylglycerol：TG
　（トリアシルグリセロール（中性脂肪））
total cholesterol：Tcho（総コレステロール）
free fatty acid：FFA（遊離脂肪酸）
phospholipid：PL（リン脂質）
ketone body, acetoaetic acid（ケトン体・アセト酢酸）
3-hydroxybutyric acid（3-ヒドロキシ酪酸）
total ketone body（総ケトン体）

The Vitamins（ビタミン類）
vitamin B_1（ビタミンB_1）
vitamin B_2（ビタミンB_2）
vitamin B_6（ビタミンB_6）
vitamin B_{12}（ビタミンB_{12}）
vitamin C（ビタミンC）
$1,25(OH)_2$ Vitamin D（$1,25(OH)_2$ビタミンD）
vitamin E（ビタミンE）

The Electrolytes, minerals, others
　（電解質，ミネラルほか）
sodium：Na（ナトリウム）
chloride：Cl（クロール）
potassium：K（カリウム）
calcium：Ca（カルシウム）
inorganic phosphate：IP（無機リン酸）
magnesium：Mg（マグネシウム）
iron：Fe（鉄(人体の)）
total iron-binding capacity：TIBC（総鉄結合能）
unsaturated iron-binding capacity：UIBC
　（不飽和鉄結合能）
copper：Cu（銅）
zinc：Zn（亜鉛）
ceruloplasmin：Cp（セルロプラスミン）
transferrin：Tf（トランスフェリン）

Liver function tests（肝機能検査）
aspartate aminotransferase：AST
　（アスパラギン酸アミノトランスフェーゼ）
　（＝glutamic oxaloacetic transferase：GOT
　（グルタミン酸オキサロ酢酸トランスアミナーゼ）
alanine transaminase：ALT
　（アラニントランスアミナーゼ）
　（＝glutamic pyruvic transaminase：GPT
　（グルタミン酸ピルビン酸トランスアミナーゼ））
alkaline phosphatase：ALP（アルカリホスファターゼ）
leucine aminopeptidase：LAT
　（ロイシンアミノペプチダーゼ）
γ-glutamyl transferase：γ-GT
　（γ-グルタミルトランスフェラーゼ）
cholinesterase：ChE（コリンエステラーゼ）
direct bilirubin：DBIL/Dbil（直接ビリルビン）
indirect bilirubin：IBIL（間接ビリルビン）

Kidney function tests（腎機能検査）
sodium thiosulfate clearance：Cthio
　（チオ硫酸ナトリウムクリアランス）
creatinine clearance：Ccr
　（クレアチニンクリアランス(24時間)）
urinary albumin（尿中アルブミン）

Pituitary function tests（下垂体機能検査）
thyroid-stimulating hormone：TSH
　（甲状腺刺激ホルモン）
growth hormone：GH（成長ホルモン）
adrenocorticotropic hormone：ACTH
　（副腎皮質刺激ホルモン）

Thyroid function tests（甲状腺機能検査）
triiodothyronine：T_3
　（トリヨードチロニン（トリヨードサイロニン））
free triiodothyronine：Free T_3
　（遊離トリヨードチロニン（遊離トリヨードサイロニン））
total thyroxin：T_4（血清総チロキシン（サイロキシン））
free thyroxin：Free T_4
　（遊離チロキシン（サイロキシン））

Pancreas, digestive tube tests
　（膵臓・消化管機能検査）
immunoreactive insulin：IRI（免疫反応性インスリン）
C-peptide：CPR（C-ペプチド）
immunoactive glucagon（免疫性グルカゴン）
secretin（セクレチン）
amylase：AMY（アミラーゼ）

Parathyroid tests（副甲状腺機能検査）
parathyroid hormone：HS-PTH（副甲状腺ホルモン）
osteocalcin（オステオカルシン）

Appendix 2
The Names of Diseases and Disorders
疾患の名称

1. The Gastroenterological System （消化器系）
1-1 Oral Cavity （口腔部）
gingivitis （歯肉炎）
glossitis （舌炎）
periodontal disease （歯周病）
   cf. chronic periodontitis （慢性歯周炎（歯槽膿漏））
pulpitis （歯髄炎）
malocclusion （不正咬合）
stomatitis （口内炎）
tooth decay （う歯）

1-2 Upper Gastrointestinal Tract （上部胃腸管）
gastric mucosal lesion (acute)：AGML
   （（急性）粘膜病変）
gastritis （胃炎）
gastroenteritis （胃腸炎）
gastroesophageal reflux disease：GERD
   （胃食道逆流疾患）
hiatal hernia （裂孔ヘルニア）
infantile colic （乳児疝痛）
peptic ulcer （消化性潰瘍）
   gastric ulcer （胃潰瘍）
   duodenal ulcer （十二指腸潰瘍）

1-3 Lower Gastrointestinal Tract （下部胃腸管）
appendicitis (acute) （（急性）虫垂炎）
abdominal hernia （腹部ヘルニア）
celiac disease (＝gluten-induced enteropathy)
   （セリアック病（グルテン過敏性腸症））
cholecystitis （胆嚢炎）
cholelithiasis （胆石症）
Crohn disease (＝regional enteritis, granulomatous
   colitis) （クローン病（限局性腸炎, 肉芽腫性大腸炎））
diverticulosis （憩室症）
hemorrhoids （痔核）
ileus （腸閉塞（病理）（イレウス））
inflammatory bowel disease （炎症性腸疾患）
irritable bowel syndrome：IBS （過敏性腸症候群）
malabsorption syndrome （吸収不良症候群）
rectal cancer （直腸がん）
ulcerative colitis （潰瘍性大腸炎）

(symptom) （症状）
constipation （便秘）
diarrhea （下痢）

1-4 Accessory Organs of Gasteroenterological System （消化器系付属緒器官）
cholelithiasis （胆石症）
cholecystitis （胆のう炎）
congenital biliary atresia （先天性胆道閉鎖症）
fatty liver (acute, chronic) （脂肪肝）
hepatitis (acute) （（急性）肝炎）
   acute viral hepatitis （急性ウイルス性肝炎）
   fulminant hepatitis （劇症肝炎）
hepatic failure （肝不全）
hepatomegaly （肝腫大）
jaundice （黄疸）
liver cirrhosis （肝硬変）
pancreatitis (acute, chronic) （膵炎（急性, 慢性））

2. The Musculoskeletal System （筋骨格系）
achillobursitis （アキレス腱滑液包炎）
amyotrophic lateral sclerosis：ALS
   （筋委縮性側索硬化症）
cervical spine injury （頸椎損傷）
corn, clavus, heloma （鶏眼(＝うおのめ)）
disk herniation （椎間板ヘルニア）
fractures （骨折）
   fatigue fracture （疲労骨折（足））
hip dislocation （股関節脱臼）
lateral curvature （脊柱側弯症）
myasthenia gravis （重症筋無力症）
muscular dystrophy （筋ジストロフィー）
muscular atrophy （筋委縮）
osteoarthritis （変形性関節症）
osteogenesis imperfecta （骨形成不全症）
osteoporosis （骨粗鬆症）
osteomalacia （骨軟化症）
osteomyelitis （骨髄症）
postmenopausal osteoporosis （閉経後骨粗鬆症）
rheumatism (＝rheumatic disease)
   （リウマチ（リウマチ性疾患））
rheumatoid arthritis：RA （関節リウマチ）
sprains （捻挫）
strains （挫傷）
temporomandibular joint disorder （顎関節症）

3. The Cardiovascular System （心臓血管系）
anemia （貧血）
   aplastic anemia （再生不良性貧血）
   autoimmune hemolytic anemia：AHA

（自己免疫性溶血性貧血）
angina pectoris （狭心症）
aplastic anemia （再生不良性貧血）
arteriosclerosis （動脈硬化症）
atherosclerosis （粥状硬化症）
atherothrombotic infarction （アテローム血栓性梗塞）
cardiac arrest （心停止）
cardiac failure （心不全）
myocarditis （心筋炎）
hemophilia （血友病）
pericarditis （心膜炎）
phlebitis （静脈炎）
hypertension （高血圧）
　　essential hypertension （本態性高血圧）
　　secondary hypertension （二次性高血圧）
ischemic heart disease （虚血性心疾患）
myocardial infarction （心筋梗塞）
sepsis （敗血症）
stroke （脳卒中）
thrombophelebitis （血栓静脈炎）
thrombosis （血栓）
valvular heart disease （心臓弁膜症）
subarachnoid hemorrhage：SAH （くも膜下出血）

4. The Nervous System （神経系）
4-1 Nerves （神経）
Alzheimer disease （アルツハイマー病）
　　senile dementia of Alzheimer type
　　　　（アルツハイマー型認知症）
brain abscess （脳膿瘍）
brain contusion （脳挫傷）
cluster headache （群発性頭痛）
epilepsy （てんかん）
Guillain-Barre syndrome （＝acute inflammatory
　demyelinating polyradiculoneuropathy）
　　（ギラン・バレー症候群（急性炎症性脱髄性多発神経
　　根ニューロパチー））
intercostal neuralgia （肋間神経痛）
meningitis （髄膜炎）
migraine （片頭痛）
multiple sclerosis （多発性硬化症）
poliomyelitis （＝infantile paralysis）
　　（ポリオ（急性灰白髄炎））
hydrocephalus, hydrocephaly （水頭症）
spinocerebellar degeneration：SCI （脊髄小脳変性症）
Parkinson disease （パーキンソン病）
Parkinson syndrome （パーキンソン症候群）
Parkinsonism （パーキンソニズム（前頭葉委縮））
spinal cord injuries （脊髄損傷）
trigeminal neuralgia （三叉神経痛）

> Notes：脳出血，脳血管障害（脳卒中），脳梗塞，
> くも膜下出血は心臓血管系に，重症筋無力症は筋・
> 骨格系に記載．

4-2 Sense Organs （感覚器官）
1) Eyes （眼）
cataract （白内障）
conjunctivitis （結膜炎）
corneal herpes （角膜ヘルペス）

dry eye syndrome （ドライアイ症候群）
　　cf. keratoconjunctivitis sicca：KCS （乾性角結膜炎））
glaucoma （緑内障）
hearing loss （聴覚障害）
hordeolum （麦粒腫）
Meniere disease （メニエール病）
optic neuritis （視神経炎）
retinopathy （網膜症（diabetic r. 糖尿病〜，
　　hypertentive r. 高血圧性〜））

2) Ears （耳）
epidemic parotitis （＝mumps）
　　（流行性耳下腺炎（おたふくかぜ．複数形で単数扱い））
deafness （＝hearing loss, hearing impairment）
　　（難聴）
　　conductive hearing impairment （伝音性難聴）
　　presbyacusis （老年性難聴）
sensorineural hearing loss （感音難聴）
　　idiopathic bilateral sensorineural hearing loss
　　　　（特発性両側性感音難聴）
　　sudden hearing loss （突発性難聴）
otitis interna （内耳炎）
otitis media (acute, chronic) （中耳炎（急性，慢性））
tympanic membrane injury （鼓膜損傷）

3) Skin （皮膚）
atopic dermatitis （アトピー性皮膚炎）
bedsore （＝pressure ulcer, pressure sore, decubitus
　ulcer）（褥瘡）
burn （熱傷）
drug eruption （＝drug rash）（薬疹）
melanoma （黒色腫・メラノーマ）
psoriasis （乾癬）
scleroderma （強皮症）
trichophytia pompholyciformis （＝athlete's foot）
　　（汗疱状白癬（水虫））
urticaria （蕁麻疹）

5. The Respiratory System （呼吸器系）
adult respiratory distress syndrome：ARDS
　　（成人型供給窮迫症候群）
asthma （喘息）
bronchial asthma （気管支喘息）
bronchitis (acute, chronic) （気管支炎（急性，慢性））
chronic obstructive pulmonary disease：COPD
　　（慢性閉塞性肺疾患）
laryngitis (acute, chronic) （喉頭炎（急性，慢性））
nosocomial pneumonia （院内肺炎）
pharyngitis (acute, chronic) （咽頭炎（急性，慢性））
pneumonia （肺炎）
　　aspiration pneumonia （誤嚥性肺炎）
　　Pneumocystis carinii pneumonia （カリニ肺炎）
pleurisy （胸膜炎（肋膜炎））
pneumonoconiosis （塵肺症）
pneumothorax （気胸）
pulmonary tuberculosis （肺結核）
pulmonary edema （肺水腫）
pulmonary embolism （肺塞栓症）
pulmonary emphysema （肺気腫）
respiratory acidosis （呼吸性アシドーシス）

respiratory alkalosis（呼吸性アルカローシス）
tonsillitis（扁桃腺炎）

6. The Kidney and Urinary System（腎・泌尿器系）
cystitis（膀胱炎）
chronic kidney disease：CKD（慢性腎臓病）
glomerulonephritis（糸球体腎炎）
hydronephrosis（水腎症）
hyperuricemia（高尿酸血症）
malignant nephrosclerosis（悪性腎硬化症）
nephritis (acute)（(急性)腎炎）
nephrotic syndrome（ネフローゼ症候群）
peripheral nephritis（末梢腎炎）
polycystic kidney（多発性嚢胞腎）
pyelonephritis（腎盂腎炎）
renal diabetes（腎性糖尿病）
renal disease (＝end-stage renal failure)
　（腎疾患(末期腎不全)）
renal failure (acute)（(急性)腎不全）
urethritis（尿道炎）

7. The Immune/lymphatic System（免疫系／リンパ系）
allergic purpura（アレルギー性紫斑病）
allergic rhinitis（アレルギー性鼻炎）
autoimmune disease（自己免疫疾患）
Hodgkin disease（ホジキン病）
lymphedema（リンパ水腫）
lymphatic sarcoma（リンパ性肉腫）
malignant lymphoma（悪性リンパ腫）
acquired immune deficiency syndrome：AIDS
　（後天性免疫不全症候群）
malignant lymphoma（悪性リンパ腫）
leukemia（白血病）
pollenosis, pollinosis（花粉症）
systemic lupus erythematosus：SLE
　（全身性エリテマトーデス）
hyperimmunoglobulin E syndrome（高IgE症候群）

8. Metabolic Disorders（代謝障害）
一般的に代謝障害は5群に分類される．
8-1 Dyslipidemia（脂質代謝異常）
hyperlipidemia（脂質異常症(高脂血症)）
fatty liver（脂肪肝）
nonalcoholic steatohepatitis：NASH
　（非アルコール性肝脂肪性肝炎）
non-alcoholic fatty liver disease：NAFLD
　（非アルコール性脂肪肝）
obesity（肥満症）
　simple obesity (primary obesity)
　　（単純性肥満(一次性肥満，原発性肥満)）
　symptomatic obesity (secondary obesity)
　　（症候性肥満(二次性肥満)）
metabolic syndrome（メタボリックシンドローム）
8-2 Saccharometabolic Disorder（糖質代謝異常）
diabetes mellitus：DM（糖尿病）
　type 1 diabetes mellitus
　　（1型糖尿病(インスリン依存型糖尿病)）
　type 2 diabetes mellitus
　　（2型糖尿病(インスリン非依存型糖尿病)）
　secondary diabetes（二次性糖尿病）
　　acromegaly（先端巨大症）
　　chronic pancreatitis（慢性膵炎）
　　chronic hepatitis（慢性肝炎）
　　cirrhosis（肝硬変）
　　Cushing disease（クッシング症候群）
　　hyperthyroidism（甲状腺機能亢進症）
　Complications（合併症）
　　diabetic neuropathy（糖尿病神経障害）
　　diabetic nephropathy（糖尿病腎症）
　　diabetic retinopathy（糖尿病性網膜症）
angiopathy（血管障害
　arteriosclerosis（動脈硬化）
　　→hypertension 高血圧，cerebral infarction 脳梗塞，
　　myocardial infarction 心筋梗塞）
glycogenosis（糖原病(inherited g. 遺伝性糖原病)）
8-3 Proteometabolic Disorder（たんぱく質代謝異常）
amyloidosis（アミロイドーシス）
carpal tunnel syndrome（手根管症候群）
hypoproteinemia（低たんぱく血症）
8-4 Uric acid Metabolic Disorder（尿酸代謝異常）
gout（痛風）
8-5 Other Metabolic Disorders（その他の代謝障害）
1) Adult Diseases（成人病）
cancerがん，strokes脳卒中，heart diseases心疾患，
　hypertension高血圧
2) Life Style-related Diseases（生活習慣病）
cerebral hemorrhage（脳出血）
cerebral infarction（脳梗塞）
hypertension（高血圧）
myocardial infarction (MI)（心筋梗塞）
chronic bronchitis（慢性気管支炎）
pulmonary emphysema（肺気腫）
pulmonary squamous cell carcinoma
　（肺扁平上皮がん）

9. Nutritonal Disease（栄養疾患）
adiposity（脂肪過多症）
beriberi（脚気）
dietary calcium deficiency（食事性カルシウム欠乏症）
dwarfism（小人症）
emaciation (＝vitamin D deficiency)
　（るいそう(ビタミンD欠乏症)）
rickets（くる病）
iron deficiency（鉄欠乏症）
kwashiorkor（クワシオルコル）
malabsorption syndrome（吸収不良症候群）
marasmus（マラスムス(栄養性消耗症)）
niacin deficiency (＝pellagra)
　（ナイアシン欠乏症(ペラグラ)）
overnutrition（過栄養）
protein-energy malnutrition：PEM
　（たんぱく質エネルギー栄養障害）
thiamin deficiency（チアミン欠乏症）
vitamin A (B, C, D, E, K) deficiency
　（ビタミンA (B, C, D, E, K) 欠乏症）

10. Mental Health（精神保健）

alcoholism（アルコール依存症）
anxiety disorders（不安障害）
Asperger syndrome（アスペルガー症候群）
autism, autistic disorder（自閉症）
dementia（認知症）
depersonalization disorder（離人症性障害）
dissociative disorder（解離性障害）
 dissociative identify disorder（解離性同一性障害）
depression（うつ病）
Down syndrome（ダウン症候群）
drug dependency（薬物依存症）
eating disorders（摂食障害）
 anorexia nervosa（神経性食欲不振症）
 bulimia nervosa（神経性大食症）
epilepsy（てんかん）
attention deficit hyperactivity disorder：ADHD
 （注意欠陥多動障害）
mental retardation（精神遅滞）
personality disorders（人格障害）
panic disorder（パニック障害）
Pick disease（ピック病）
schizophrenia（統合失調症）
substance abuse（物質乱用）

11. The Endocrine System（内分泌系（ホルモンの病気））

Addioson disease（＝primary chronic adrenocortical insufficiency）
 （アジソン病（原発性慢性副腎機能低下症））
Basedow disease（＝Graves disease）
 （バセドウ病（グレーブス病））
Cushing disease（クッシング病）
diabetes mellitus（真性糖尿病）
diabetes insipidus（尿崩症）
gigantism（巨人症）
hyperthyroidism（甲状腺機能亢進症）
hypothyroidism（甲状腺機能低下症）
thyroiditis（甲状腺炎）

12. The Reproductive System（生殖系）

amenorrhea（無月経症）
candidiasis (candidosis)（カンジダ症）
Chlamydia infections（クラミジア感染症）
dysmenorrhea（月経困難症）
endometriosis（子宮内膜症）
gonorrhea（淋病）
infertility（不妊症）
 climacteric disturbance（＝menopausal syndrome）（更年期障害）
pregnancy-induced hypertension（妊娠高血圧症候群）
prostatitis（前立腺炎）
prostatic hyperplasia（前立腺肥大症）
premenstrual syndrome（月経前症候群）
syphilis（梅毒）
trichomoniasis（トリコモナス症）
uterine myoma, hysteromyoma（子宮筋腫）

13. Infectious Disease（感染病）

bacterial food poisoning（細菌性食中毒）
cholera（コレラ）
cold（風邪）
diphtheria（ジフテリア）
Enterobacterial infection（腸内細菌感染症）
enterobiasis（蟯虫症）
herpes zoster（帯状疱疹）
hemorrhagic fever（出血熱）
HIV (human immunodeficiency virus) infection
 （ヒト免疫不全ウイルス感染症＝AIDS）
influenza (flu)（インフルエンザ）
 H1N1 influenza（H1N1インフルエンザ）
Norovirus infection（ノロウイルス感染症）
pneumococcal infection（肺炎球菌感染症）
rheumatic fever（リウマチ熱）
Rickettsia infection（リケッチア感染症）
Salmonella infection（サルモネラ菌感染症）
severe acute respiratory syndrome：SARS
 （重症急性呼吸器症候群）
staphylococcal infection（ブドウ球菌感染症）
tetanus（破傷風）
typhoid fever（腸チフス）
toxoplasmosis（トキソプラズマ症）

著者紹介

清水　雅子（しみず　まさこ）
1982年　岡山大学大学院教育学研究科英語教育専攻修士課程修了
　　　　元川崎医療福祉大学医療福祉学部／大学院医療福祉学研究科
　　　　教授，元北里大学非常勤講師
著　書　「医療技術者のための医学英語入門」(1991)，「病気の英語入門」(1994)，「はじめての栄養英語」(2007)，「医療従事者のための医学英語入門」(2011) 以上講談社，「ドーランド図説医学大辞典第28版」(1997, 分担執筆) 廣川書店，「福祉・介護系学生のための総合英語」(2007) 南雲堂，「講義録医学英語Ⅰ」(2005, 編集)，「リハビリテーション英語の基本用語と表現」(2015)，「リハビリテーションの基礎英語改訂第3版」(2017) 以上メジカルビュー社，「PT・OT・STのための国際学会はじめの一歩」(2014) 三輪書店．

J. パトリック バロン
1969年　University of Pennsylvania
1975年　The Doctorial Program at University of London: School of Oriental and African Studies（PhD.ABD）
　　　　聖マリアンナ医科大学助教授を経て，東京医科大学 名誉教授
著　書　「医師のための診療英会話」(2002, 共著)，「講義録医学英語Ⅲ」(2006)，「医学英語活用辞典」(2012, 総監訳) 以上メジカルビュー社，「医学英語コミュニケーション1」「同2」「同3」(2003, 共著) 以上朝倉書店．

NDC 590　121p　26 cm

はじめての臨床栄養英語（りんしょうえいようえいご）

2013年 3月30日　第1刷発行
2022年 2月18日　第5刷発行

著　者　清水雅子・J. パトリック バロン
発行者　髙橋明男
発行所　株式会社　講談社
　　　　〒112-8001　東京都文京区音羽2-12-21
　　　　　販　売　(03)5395-4415
　　　　　業　務　(03)5395-3615
編　集　株式会社　講談社サイエンティフィク
　　　　代表　堀越俊一
　　　　〒162-0825　東京都新宿区神楽坂2-14 ノービィビル
　　　　　編　集　(03)3235-3701
印刷所　株式会社双文社印刷
製本所　株式会社国宝社

落丁本・乱丁本は，購入書店名を明記のうえ，講談社業務宛にお送りください．送料小社負担にてお取替えします．なお，この本の内容についてのお問い合わせは講談社サイエンティフィク宛にお願いいたします．
定価はカバーに表示してあります．

© Masako Shimizu and J. Patrick Barron, 2013

本書のコピー，スキャン，デジタル化等の無断複製は著作権法上での例外を除き禁じられています．本書を代行業者等の第三者に依頼してスキャンやデジタル化することはたとえ個人や家庭内の利用でも著作権法違反です．

JCOPY　〈(社)出版者著作権管理機構 委託出版物〉
複写される場合は，その都度事前に，(社)出版者著作権管理機構（電話03-5244-5088, FAX 03-5244-5089, e-mail：info@jcopy.or.jp）の許諾を得てください．

Printed in Japan

ISBN978-4-06-155621-8

講談社の科学英語

はじめての栄養英語
えっ、Dietって、やせるって意味じゃないの?
栄養士の私はDietitianなんだ!
美味しく学べる英語のスキル

清水 雅子・著
B5・108頁・定価1,980円(税込)

やさしい英文で初学者でも栄養英語に親しめるよう工夫されたテキスト。栄養素、代謝、解剖生理、消化吸収、食品添加物、食物アレルギーなどを、やさしく短い英文でとりあげた。

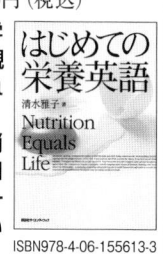

ISBN978-4-06-155613-3

医療従事者のための医学英語入門
清水 雅子・著
A5・213頁・定価2,750円(税込)

人体組織、器官を中心に基礎医学をコンパクトに収載した1991年刊の好評テキスト『医療技術者のための医学英語入門』が新版となって登場。図版も追加され、さらに使いやすく!コメディカルの養成校向けテキストに最適。

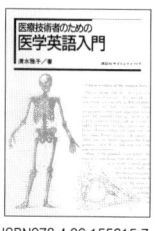

ISBN978-4-06-155615-7

英文ニュースで学ぶ健康とライフスタイル
田中 芳文・編著
B5・110頁・定価2,860円(税込)

医療や健康の話題を扱ったニュース記事で英語リーディング能力をレベルアップ!一般人向けの記事だから、出てくる用語は一般常識レベルで、文章も読みやすい。看護系や健康栄養系の学生のための新しい英語トレーニング!

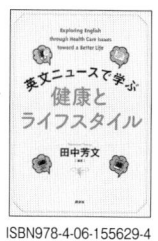

ISBN978-4-06-155629-4

やさしい英語ニュースで学ぶ現代社会と健康
田中 芳文・編著
B5・110頁・定価2,640円(税込)

医療、福祉、栄養系など健康と深くかかわる学生のための教科書。とくに現代社会とのかかわりを意識させる英語ニュースをピックアップ。一般向けニュースだからスラスラ読める。

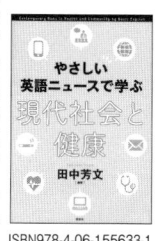

ISBN978-4-06-155633-1

はじめての薬学英語
野口 ジュディー／神前 陽子／スミス 朋子／天ヶ瀬 葉子・著
CD付き
B5・103頁・定価2,750円(税込)

扱っている英文は薬学に直結する内容。アメリカ厚生労働省の市民向け健康ウェブサイトや高校の生物学教科書など、専門知識がなくても簡単に読めるものばかり。分量も半期の授業で難なくこなせるように配慮。

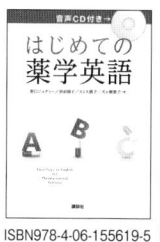

ISBN978-4-06-155619-5

Judy先生の耳から学ぶ科学英語
CD付き
野口 ジュディー・著
B5・92頁・定価3,740円(税込)

数式の分数や乗数、単位や尺度、多用される器具機械の名称や操作用語、基礎的な化学名などの広い分野の科学英語をCDの模範発音を聞きながら理解できる1冊。

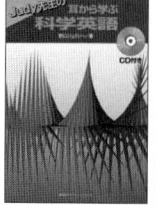

ISBN978-4-06-153937-2

耳から学ぶ楽しいナース英語
中西 睦子・監修 野口 ジュディー／川越 栄子／仁平 雅子・著
B5・110頁・定価3,740円(税込)

CDを聞きながら学ぶ看護英語の決定版。国際化時代の医療現場では英語は不可欠の時代、聞きとれること話せることは必須要素。「どうかしましたか」「どのように痛みますか」こんな会話が話せるようになる1冊。

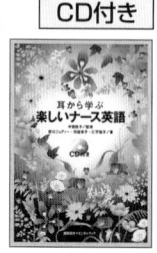

CD付き

ISBN978-4-06-153672-2

英語で読む21世紀の健康
阿部 祚子／正木 美知子・著
B5・102頁・定価1,980円(税込)

健康・栄養・福祉についてWHOから発信される的確ですぐれた英文を選りすぐり、わかりやすい解説をつけ健康科学系の大学・短大などへ向けた画期的な英語の教科書。

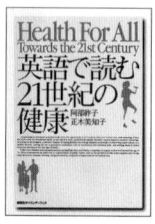

ISBN978-4-06-153664-7

Let's Study English! Health and Nutrition
英語で読む健康と栄養
横尾 信男・編著
A5・94頁・定価1,650円(税込)

栄養系学生のための教養課程英語テキスト。健康な食生活に必要な知識(栄養素やその摂取法、病気にならない食生活・エクササイズ、酒やタバコの害、食中毒、ストレス解消など)を幅広く学べるよう編集。

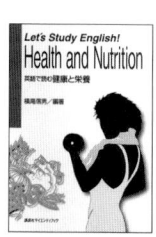

ISBN978-4-06-153951-8

※表示価格は消費税(10%)が加算されています。

講談社サイエンティフィク　https://www.kspub.co.jp/

「2022年2月10日現在」

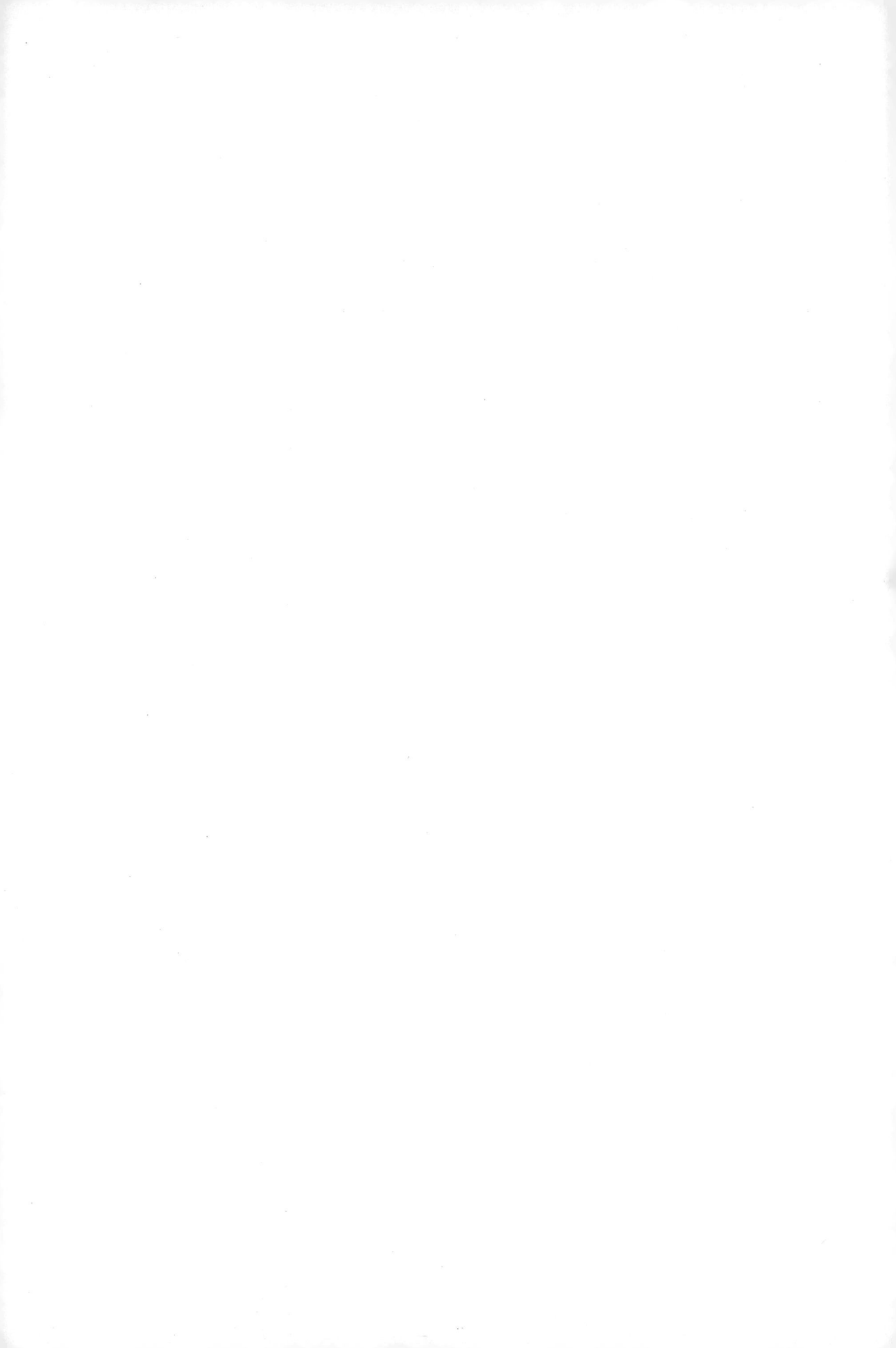